PUSH

TRY US TODAY!

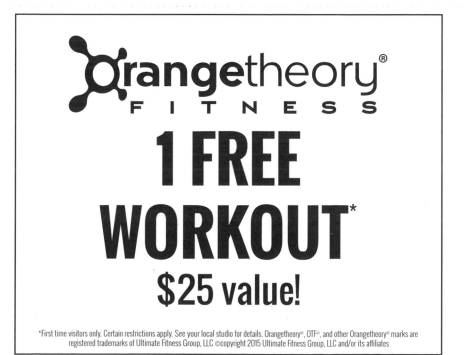

** Orangetheory® FITNESS**

1 FREE WORKOUT*

$25 value!

*First time visitors only. Certain restrictions apply. See your local studio for details. Orangetheory®, OTF®, and other Orangetheory® marks are registered trademarks of Ultimate Fitness Group, LLC ©copyright 2015 Ultimate Fitness Group, LLC and/or its affiliates

---

Ợrangetheory® FITNESS

1 FREE WORKOUT*

$25 value!

*First time visitors only. Certain restrictions apply. See your local studio for details. Orangetheory®, OTF®, and other Orangetheory® marks are registered trademarks of Ultimate Fitness Group, LLC ©copyright 2015 Ultimate Fitness Group, LLC and/or its affiliates

TRY US TODAY!

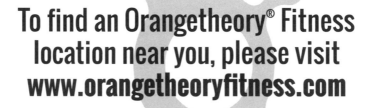

To find an Orangetheory® Fitness
location near you, please visit
www.orangetheoryfitness.com

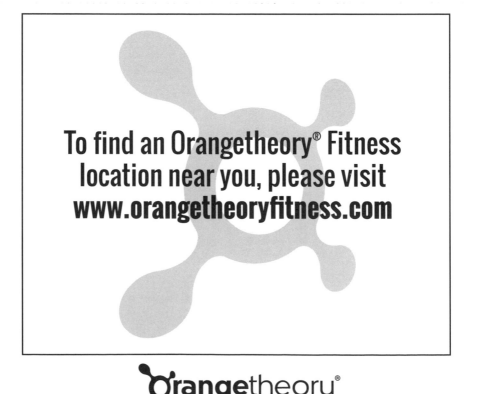

To find an Orangetheory® Fitness
location near you, please visit
www.orangetheoryfitness.com

orangetheory®
F I T N E S S

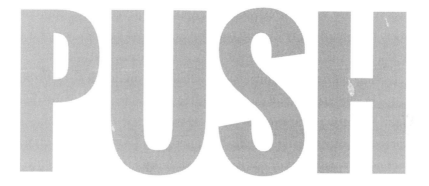

PUSH

A Guide to Living an All Out Life: The Story of Orangetheory® Fitness

ELLEN LATHAM, MS

Foreword by
BRENDON AYANBADEJO
Orangetheory Fitness Area Developer/Franchisee
Former NFL player (Miami Dolphins, Chicago Bears, Baltimore Ravens)

Ultimate Fitness Group, LLC ■ Fort Lauderdale, FL

Published by
Ultimate Fitness Group, LLC
Fort Lauderdale, FL

Publisher's Cataloging-in-Publication Data
Latham, Ellen.

Push : a guide to living an all out life, the story of Orangetheory Fitness / by Ellen Latham. – Fort Lauderdale, FL : Ultimate Fitness Group, LLC, 2015.

p. ; cm.

ISBN13: 978-0-9980015-0-0

1. Physical fitness. 2. Physical education and training. I. Title.

GV481.L37 2015
613.7—dc23   2015948636

Project coordination by Jenkins Group, Inc.
www.BookPublishing.com

Interior design by Brooke Camfield

Printed in the United States of America
19 18 17 16 15 • 5 4 3 2 1

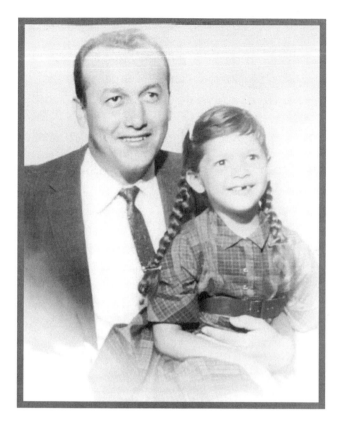

To my dad,
the wind beneath my wings

Contents

Foreword

As a former professional athlete, I believe I came out of the womb with a ball, jump rope, or dumbbell in hand. Since I was a kid, I've tried every fitness concept under the sun. I've even created some of my own fitness programming. At one time or another I've done diving, junior lifeguards, wrestling, jujitsu, climbing, hiking, mountain biking, track, baseball, football, basketball, CrossFit, Pilates, P90X, Tae Bo, triathlons, tennis, surfing—you name it. Anything fun and fitness related under the sun and I am all in.

With that being said, my fitness appetite and palate are quite sophisticated. Now don't get me wrong: you can take the most boring, bland workout—like doing burpees for 20 minutes straight—and it's going to be the hardest workout of your life. But how do you create a fitness concept that is not only challenging but also fun and engaging? On top of that, how do you create a group mentality so that even the weakest in the pack are able to succeed and exceed their own expectations without slowing down the leaders of the pack?

That is exactly what Ellen Latham did when she created Orangetheory Fitness. At Orangetheory, you have high-level athletes, and you have sedentary individuals who want to get in the best shape of their lives. You throw them all into a little room with loud music and all the necessary fitness tools to challenge strength, endurance, power, proprioceptive capabilities, coordination, and athleticism. What happens next? Amazing results.

On February 3, 2013, I was playing in what would be not only my last game as a Baltimore Raven but also my last as a professional football player. It was Super Bowl XLVII, and my team was playing against the San Francisco 49ers. That Super Bowl is infamously known for the 20-minute blackout that occurred during the second half of the game and delayed our victory for 20 minutes. After the game, I told myself I was going to stay in bed and soak up the championship for two weeks. I'd just spent 30 straight weeks playing football and had achieved a lifelong goal!

While that was my plan, it was not my wife's or Orangetheory's. On Wednesday morning, February 6, at about 9:00, I kept hearing my wife, Natalee, say, "Wake up! We're going to go work out." The little voice in my head kept saying, "Wait! I've got 11 more days!" Let's just say that didn't exactly work out in my favor. Five minutes later, I was in the car on my way to my very first Orangetheory Fitness class.

When I started doing Orangetheory, I immediately fell in love with the workout because it is a completely different take on fitness. Orangetheory is fitness from the inside out. It starts with your heart—the strongest muscle in your body. As a professional athlete, you know there are certain things you want to work on aside from your sports skills. You need endurance so you can perform at a high level play after play. You need strength so you can be stronger than your opponents. You also need to be fast, so you work on power and explosive ability.

You develop all of those abilities—endurance, strength, and power—at Orangetheory, but you also use the five-zone interval training to ensure that you're working out at the appropriate intensity. The OTbeat heart rate–monitoring system lets you see how rested or fatigued you are so you can perform at your best at any particular point of the workout. You know how hard you're working, which helps reduce the risk of injury, and you know when you can push yourself. I love having the ability to see that real-time biofeedback.

Since I've been involved with Orangetheory, I've run my fastest mile ever at 5:20. I'm now a very competent indoor water rower and have set personal bests rowing 2,000 meters and 500 meters. I was introduced to rowing via Orangetheory and world champion rower Josh Crosby, who's on the company's Fitness Advisory Board. I have had the honor of going head to head against Josh on several occasions. Let's just say we have to bolt the water rowers down when we get lined up next to each other!

While I am in a different kind of shape than I was when I played pro football, at 39 I am arguably in better shape now than I ever have been in my entire life! Just last week I ran my personal best three-mile time at 19:30. That's a 6:30/mile pace, which is 100 percent attributed to my training at Orangetheory. In fact, in 2008—the height of my NFL career—I competed against my agent, Drew Rosenhaus, in a three-mile race. I finished in 23 minutes, and he finished in 24 minutes. Eight years later, I have dropped my time by 3 minutes and 30 seconds!

Orangetheory Fitness has been a life-changing experience. And if it could change my life as a professional athlete, what can it do for all the fitness enthusiasts out there and the people who are scared to take that next step to control their health and fitness and get in shape? After I had been a member for a couple of months, the lightbulb went off in my head. I knew this would be a huge opportunity for me to continue my life in the fitness arena, not as a professional athlete but as a fitness franchise owner. I decided to take the next step and look into franchising. I still lived in Florida during the offseason, going back to my days with the Miami Dolphins. I became an Orangetheory franchisee and was immediately welcomed with open arms into the Orangetheory family. Lucky man that I am, my wife and our two children were born in Fort Lauderdale. Now my second career was also conceived in Fort Lauderdale, Florida!

When Ellen asked me to write this foreword, I was honored and immediately agreed. I think you'll enjoy learning about how Orangetheory was created and why it's so effective, as well as getting to know Ellen, who is a force of nature. She has so many amazing attributes, but one that really pops out at me is her energy. She is the essence of the color orange, a color that is associated with happiness and enthusiasm. She has inspired thousands of people, including me. I think she'll inspire you, too.

In an ever-changing business, I am ultimately impressed with Ellen's ability to stay ahead of the fitness curve. The Orangetheory workout is the ultimate proof of her intelligence, drive, and vision—the concept is 10 years ahead of any other fitness product out there. Enjoy the journey that Ellen is about to take you on! It is a fascinating one.

Brendon Ayanbadejo
Orangetheory Fitness Area Developer/Franchisee
Former NFL player (Miami Dolphins, Chicago Bears, Baltimore Ravens)

Acknowledgments

Before you read about how to Push your oxygen intake, I would like to acknowledge some of the most important people who have oxygenated my life. First and foremost, I thank my mother and father, Rose and Arthur Calandrelli, for the secure, loving family base that you both created in my life. Mom, your intense belief in me and your deep love have kept me strong. Dad, you were the strongest person—both inside and out—I've ever met. I'm blessed to be your daughter.

I am also grateful for the love of my brothers and sisters and their families—my older brother, Arthur Calandrelli, and his husband, my brother-in-law, Ismael Martinez; my sister, Cindy, and brother-in-law, John Teeto, and their sons, Johnny, Nicholas, and Michael; and my younger brother, Chris Calandrelli, and sister-in-law, Shirley. You all know that family is everything to me.

To my son, Evan Latham—you are the best thing I ever created! You are so smart and have taught me so much. I've loved watching you become a focused, excited, and caring young man. Congratulations on co-owning two very successful Orangetheory franchises. Thank you, Holly, my new daughter-in-law, for loving and supporting my most prized possession.

To Nick Granteed, my partner in life—you are my rock! You have always believed in me, even when there were moments I did not. I am lucky to have you in my life. I love you!

Thanks to my dear friends Jackie and Al Fernandez for your constant support and encouragement. Special thanks to Sue Sausmer, my manager, and Casey Librizzi, my fitness manager at Ellen's Ultimate Workout, for maintaining five-star service while I have been on my Orange journey. I'm also grateful for some true friends—Roxanne Madio, Patti Williams, Jeannine Reylet, Megan Wachtstetter, and Jennifer O'Neill. Thank you for your love and support.

Thank you to Kelly James-Enger. You were a complete joy to work with and exactly the person I needed to get my material on paper and capture my voice.

I give special thanks to my partners—Dave Long, Jerome Kern, and Dave Hardy. There is a lot of testosterone floating around here, but you have always treated me with respect and as an equal. You are visionaries with a commitment to excellence, and it has been an exhilarating ride! Thank you.

Thank you to the Orangetheory corporate team, especially Chan Gannaway, Barb Moylan, Corey Summers ("Hawk"), Clara Assasel, Jhoel Gaona, and John Driscoll, for collaborating and supporting my fitness vision (and keeping all pens away from me).

To all of the area reps and franchisees, thank you for the commitment you have made. I am so excited to be on this journey with you.

With intense gratitude, I thank all members of Orangetheory Fitness studios for choosing this training method. The ultimate desire I have is for *you* to "live in the best version of you"!

Section 1

About Orangetheory:
A Fitness Formula for Results

1

It's Not You—
It's Your Workout

Splat!

That's the sound of a fat cell exploding.

What does that have to do with fitness? Everything.

Most people exercise because they want to "splat" the fat cell. They just don't call it that. They join the gym because they're overweight. They're out of shape. They want to lose their baby weight. They had a health scare. They have a high school reunion coming up . . . a long-awaited vacation . . . a wedding. Or they just don't feel very good.

What they say is that they want to get in shape.

But what they *really* want is to splat the fat cells. And to become, as I say, a **metabolically charged body**.

You've Been Doing It Wrong

It's certainly not the lack of knowledge.

In 40+ years in the fitness industry, I've never met anyone who didn't know that you're supposed to work out. The fitness industry is big business—health clubs alone netted more than $22 billion in 2013. (And that's not counting home workout programs or the equipment—think running shoes, tennis racquets, golf clubs—we buy to get and stay in shape!) About 50 million Americans are members of gyms and health clubs, and millions more exercise at home or outdoors. Yet despite what we know we should do, studies show that only 20 percent of adults get the recommended amount of cardiovascular and strength exercise the Centers for Disease Control and Prevention recommend.

In fact, at a typical gym, by year's end nearly half of its members will have given up and abandoned their gym memberships.

So, something is wrong.

Obviously, if you don't work out, you're not going to see results. But what if you do exercise? You may have been inspired by a toned, lean body you saw in a magazine, or on Instagram, or in a television commercial. You were sold a promise—a promise that if you work out, you'll achieve that body. It's become an art in advertising to sell us on that perfect body.

But for most of us, that promise fails to come true. While exercise—any kind of exercise—is good for you, the vast majority of everyday exercisers don't get the results they want.

Their workouts don't work.

Why? The answer is one word: intensity. Actually, lack of it.

Most people just don't work out hard enough. They don't have a systematic approach to their training. They turn on a treadmill and go into a mindless state for 30, 40, 60 minutes. Then they wonder why that time on the treadmill isn't changing their body.

It's because they didn't splat the fat.

Hey, *something* is better than *nothing*. Walk and you'll improve your overall health. But you won't change the shape of your body or get a leaner, stronger, more efficient fat-burning body, a **highly metabolically charged body.** To do that, you must exercise in a very different way (more about that in a bit).

Gyms Don't Work

The fact is that gyms don't work for many people, especially deconditioned, unknowledgeable members. Gyms are full of metal machines and confusing-looking apparatuses. Once you join, your workout is up to you. That's the gym model. But few people know how to create a results-oriented exercise program. So they give up.

Most workouts don't work for the following reasons:

Lack of a program. When you join a typical gym, you're on your own. If you're a woman, you probably wind up on the elliptical or treadmill, thinking that cardio is the answer. If you're a guy, you grab dumbbells and try to build some muscle.

But it's all guesswork. You're flying by the seat of your pants. When you want mega results, you can't fly by the seat of your pants. You need focus and an effective program—but you probably don't know how to put together an effective program.

Improper form. Most people at gyms use weight machines instead of free weights because the former are easier to use. But unless you know how to set each machine for your body, you may use it improperly. And if you don't know how to lift weights, using poor form will prevent results and may cause injury.

Imbalanced routine. Not to sound sexist, but women like cardio. Guys like to lift weights. The problem is that women wind up doing nothing but cardio, and guys do nothing but lift weights! A true fitness routine includes cardiovascular exercise, strength training for what I call "inside" and "outside" muscles, and power training. Almost no one does all of that at the gym or at home.

Women think cardio will help them burn fat and give them great bodies. They don't understand muscle overload and that creating more muscle on the body is what burns calories. Likewise, the guys wanting big arms or a carved chest don't realize that the heart is a muscle. If the body is to work as a machine, that muscle has to be worked as well, just like the chest muscles and biceps muscles.

Undertraining. This is probably the biggest reason workouts don't work. People don't realize that to train the body, you have to challenge it, particularly with cardio. You have to push yourself, and most people don't do that on their own. Take 40-year-old Marilyn, who had been exercising since her 20s. Marilyn typically took five classes a week, yet she never got the results she was looking for. While she was working out a lot, she was actually undertraining because she never worked out hard enough. Now, she spends three hours a week at Orangetheory Fitness (which you'll hear lots more about!) and walks around in the body she always wanted.

Overtraining. Overtraining is another reason your workout may not work. A couple of weeks ago, my 20-year-old nephew, Nicky, came home from college and was training with his friend Joe at the gym. Nicky performed Joe's weight-training routine and couldn't move for four days afterward. Obviously, Joe's routine wasn't the ideal workout for Nicky. Joe had built up to that level of training; Nicky had not. Most people, however, don't know how hard they can push themselves without overdoing it.

Plateauing. Most people do the same exercise routine over and over. That's the problem—if you don't mix it up, you'll plateau, or stop seeing results. Keep repeating the same five exercises, for example, and you may feel a sense of accomplishment when you're done, but your body isn't going to change. And plateauing happens rather quickly—in about six weeks.

Boredom. Lack of time is the number one reason people give for not exercising. Lack of results is another, but you can't discount boredom. Think about it. If you exercise regularly (or even occasionally), when was the last time you were really excited to work out? Or anticipating the rush or the satisfaction you'd have at the end of your workout session? If you said "pretty much never," you've tapped into another huge reason why gyms don't work for most of us.

The Power of a Trainer

Hey, I don't want to pooh-pooh the gym. Gyms are a great place to get some exercise, and any kind of movement is good for the body. A gym can be a great place to start, depending on your priorities. If your number one priority is to lose some weight, starting to exercise will probably help. But what about when your priorities change? Maybe you want to get more toned, or look leaner, or build a stronger body that's going to serve you well as you age. None of that is going to happen with a typical workout at the gym or at home. You need that **metabolically charged** body.

Traditional gyms do work for a few people. The people with the bodies you've admired at your fitness center have figured out the proper training—for them. Like my nephew found out, that doesn't mean it will work for you.

The other people who get results work with personal trainers. Trainers know how bodies work. A certified personal trainer has learned about the energy systems of the body and how to muscle overload properly and can put together a program for you. Trainers also educate and teach proper form and how to do the physical skills necessary to change your body. A good trainer pushes you to work harder than you would on your own.

So why don't we all have personal trainers? First of all, it's expensive. Ideally, to train the body for results, you have to do it two or three times a week, and at $75+/hour a week, you're now talking $600–$900/month to dedicate to your body. Most people can't afford that.

Personal trainers can be intimidating, too. When you're out of shape, do you really want some flawless body telling you what you need to do? Some people are inspired by a super-fit body, but others feel uncomfortable and won't even consider using a trainer.

Finally, every personal trainer has his or her own style. Some love free weights, while others have clients do a lot of body weight exercises.

Trainers often create programs for clients based on how they like to train, not necessarily what clients really need. That's called "trainer-focused" training as opposed to "client-focused" training.

An Exercise Multivitamin

So, gyms don't work, and trainers may not work—or you may not be able to afford them. What's the answer, then? That's what I wanted to find out.

I've spent my entire career in the fitness industry. My bachelor's degree is in physical education, and my master's degree is in exercise physiology. I've worked with thousands of clients and club members and have done just about every type of workout that's out there. Over the years, I obtained certifications in everything from Spinning to Pilates. I've taught step aerobics, aqua aerobics, and kickboxing classes and led running clubs and nearly any class you can do on the aerobics floor at the gym. I've spent my career educating myself about fitness and the human body.

Fitness—and helping people become stronger, healthier, and happier—is my passion. I wanted to learn everything I can about physiology—about the energy systems of the body, muscle overload, psychology, group exercise, personal training, motivation, heart rate training, training intensity, workout design. Over the past 15 years, I looked for the perfect metabolic training workout, one that had all of the elements you need to metabolically charge the body—to make the body an efficient fat burner for life.

I found elements here and there, but I never found the perfect workout. It's almost like a Pilates workout was vitamin A, a Spinning class might be vitamin E, and a high-intensity interval workout would be vitamin B6. But I couldn't find that **magic multivitamin that would give you everything you need**.

So I decided to create my own. (You'll learn more about how I created the Orangetheory Fitness workout, and how it evolved, in chapter 2.) What I originally called Ellen's Ultimate Workout is now the Orangetheory workout, an hour-long session at a studio that includes four vital elements:

- **Cardiovascular interval training.** I created three intensities of training: Base (a sustainable effort that you can maintain for 20–30 minutes); Push, where you up your intensity for a short period of time (less than three minutes); and All Out, where you up your intensity even higher but never for longer than one minute. The training model is based on five-zone heart rate training:

  - **Zone 1**, the Gray Zone. This is the very light-activity zone. You get healthier in this zone but not fitter.
  - **Zone 2**, the Blue Zone. This is the warm-up zone, which prepares you for higher-intensity exercise and a higher rate of fat release.
  - **Zone 3**, the Green Zone. This is your Base pace. It's a challenging, doable pace that you can maintain for 20–30 minutes.

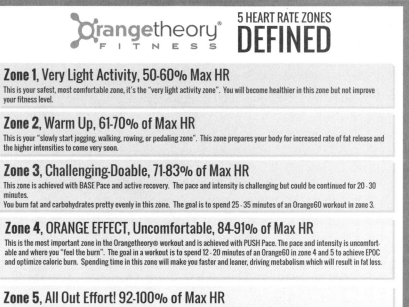

Orangetheory FITNESS · 5 HEART RATE ZONES **DEFINED**

Zone 1, Very Light Activity, 50-60% Max HR
This is your safest, most comfortable zone, it's the "very light activity zone". You will become healthier in this zone but not improve your fitness level.

Zone 2, Warm Up, 61-70% of Max HR
This is your "slowly start jogging, walking, rowing, or pedaling zone". This zone prepares your body for increased rate of fat release and the higher intensities to come very soon.

Zone 3, Challenging-Doable, 71-83% of Max HR
This zone is achieved with BASE Pace and active recovery. The pace and intensity is challenging but could be continued for 20 - 30 minutes.
You burn fat and carbohydrates pretty evenly in this zone. The goal is to spend 25 - 35 minutes of an Orange60 workout in zone 3.

Zone 4, ORANGE EFFECT, Uncomfortable, 84-91% of Max HR
This is the most important zone in the Orangetheory® workout and is achieved with PUSH Pace. The pace and intensity is uncomfortable and where you "feel the burn". The goal in a workout is to spend 12 - 20 minutes of an Orange60 in zone 4 and 5 to achieve EPOC and optimize caloric burn. Spending time in this zone will make you faster and leaner, driving metabolism which will result in fat loss.

Zone 5, All Out Effort! 92-100% of Max HR
This is the highest zone you might achieve when you empty your tank with an All Out effort. You do not need to reach this zone to experience maximum results. If you do reach this zone, you will only want to be here for 30 seconds - 1 minute at a time.

- **Zone 4**, the Orange Zone. This is your Push and the zone you want to reach during every Orangetheory workout. This is your uncomfortable zone, and it's no longer than three minutes.
- **Zone 5**, the Red Zone. This is your All Out effort; this is a very uncomfortable effort, and it's no longer than a minute.

During an Orangetheory workout, you warm up and then spend the majority of your time in the Green Zone (about 25–35 minutes) and 12–20 minutes in the Orange (and sometimes Red) Zone. We call those minutes in the Orange and Red Zones Splat Points. This type of interval training harnesses the power of EPOC, or excess postexercise oxygen consumption. That fancy phrase simply means that your body revs its metabolism so high during the workout that you continue to burn extra calories (think of splatting those fat cells) for up to 24–36 hours after your workout. I'll get into the science of the workout in chapter 3, but for now all you need to know is that this part of the workout is designed to make you a more efficient fat burner. (See Sidebar, "Build Your Fleet of Taxicabs," for a brief explanation of how this works.)

- **Strength training for outside muscles** that includes dumbbells, medicine balls, steps, and other small equipment. Cardio comprises only half of the hour-long workout because it's only half of the picture. To create that metabolically charged body, you need more than cardio. You must create more muscle. Free weights and body weight training are the most efficient way to fire all three types of muscle fibers to create and maintain the lean muscle that keeps you strong, toned, and healthy.

- **Strengthening inside muscles** using TRX straps. I've taught Pilates for years, and one of the things I love about it is that it helps strengthen your inside muscles. You may not see these muscles in the mirror, but they're literally the foundation of your body—the ones that hold the spine up and keep your shoulders back and your pelvis in a neutral position. Your ability to move starts with these unseen but essential muscles.

- **Power training** using water rowers. Rowing offers nonimpact, full-body strength and power. It increases dynamic range of motion by using one integrated motion of legs, trunk, and arms.

Build Your Fleet of Taxicabs with Base, Push, and All Out

When I talk about how the Orangetheory workout works at a cellular level to splat fat cells, I often use an analogy of having a fleet of taxicabs. Those taxicabs are your capillaries, and they're responsible for getting oxygen to the mitochondria, the tiny power plants, or engines, that fuel your body's cells. The more capillaries you have—the more taxicabs you have—the more oxygen you can deliver and the more power those mitochondria can produce. The more powerful the cells' engines are, the more calories you burn, and the more food you can metabolize, and the more fat cells go SPLAT.

When you first start working out, you may be deconditioned and have just a few taxicabs. As you start to work out in Base, you start adding a few more cabs. But it's in Push that you really build your fleet. Push is the key. That's when you really start creating more capillaries and adding more cabs to your fleet. In All Out, you add a few more.

So these little taxicabs put oxygen in and race it to the power plants to keep them burning, burning, burning. As you build your Base, you start to add a few more cabs and a few more drivers. After a few months of Base, Push, and All Out, maybe you have a huge fleet of taxicabs—all running oxygen to those power plants that are burning all the time, incinerating calories, and splatting those fat cells.

In short:

More capillaries = more oxygen delivered = more powerful cellular engines = more calories burned = more fat cells go SPLAT.

That's what happens when you train in the Orange and Red Zones, and that's what creates that metabolically charged body.

What Makes Orangetheory Different?

Now that you have an idea of what the Orangetheory workout looks like— and it sounds fun, right?—let's talk about what makes Orangetheory unlike any other exercise program out there. (I'll cover the science behind what makes it better in more detail in chapter 3.)

- **Proven research.** Orangetheory is based on science and interval-training concepts from as far back as the 1930s. I drew on two methods of exercise stimulus to create the Orangetheory workout. The first is quantitative, referring to intensity and resistance. The second is qualitative, which means changing exercises to challenge the body's neural and structural components to adapt to a new movement pattern. Orangetheory's ESP (Endurance/Strength/Power) system varies the workout from endurance-based exercise, to strength-based exercise, to power-based exercise, to combined ESP-based exercise. The results from performing it are based on EPOC, excess postoxygen consumption.

- **Efficiency.** I designed the Orangetheory workout to give you everything your body needs in just an hour. And you have to do the Orangetheory workout only two or three times a week for measureable results. **Every day is a full-body workout that's designed to hit every aspect of fitness and to challenge the human body**

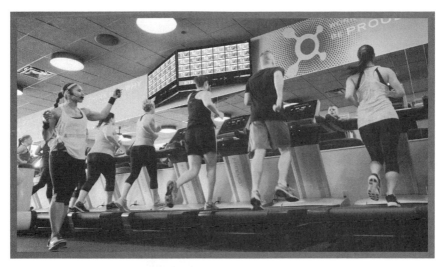

Every Orangetheory workout is a full-body workout.

as a whole. If you hired me as a personal trainer to metabolically charge your body, I'd make sure that you did cardio intervals, worked your inside and outside muscles, and did power moves every workout. Most trainers, I have to say, don't do that, and neither do other group workouts. Orangetheory does.

- **Measurability.** You can't improve what you don't measure. With Orangetheory, you're tracking your heart rate during the entire workout. You can literally see how hard your body is working by looking at the OTbeat screen, or heart rate training screen, on the wall. Your training zones are based on *your* level of fitness, and you can measure your improvement over time as you see your VO_2 max (an indicator of overall cardiovascular fitness) improve. It's not just that you *feel* like you're becoming more metabolically charged—it's not just that you look like you're getting fitter—you've got the data to prove it.

- **Intensity.** The whole Orangetheory training model is based on **training at the right intensity for the right amount of time.**

This prevents overtraining and undertraining and lets you train at what we call manageable intensity, which is the key to fitness.

- **It's for everyone.** I wanted to create a workout that anyone who wanted to try it could do. Orangetheory offers "options" (I never use the word "modifications"—it's off-putting for someone who may be deconditioned or have physical limitations). So if you want to walk, you walk. If you want to jog, you jog. If you want to run, you run. You could be a deconditioned middle-aged mom who's walking at 3.5 mph on the treadmill next to a triathlete who's sprinting at 12 mph—and you're both working in your target zones! The Orangetheory workout is based on the five heart rate training zones that apply to everyone, regardless of gender, age, and fitness level.

- **No thinking necessary.** We're living in an overstimulated world. Your brain is thinking and checking and evaluating and multitasking and just going, going, going on overload all day long. *You're* on overload. You don't want to have to think about your workout, or worry about sets, reps, how much weight to lift, or what to do first. At Orangetheory, you don't have to think. All you have to do is show up and turn off—or as I like to say, **turn off your brain to turn on your body**.

- **Coaching.** Every Orangetheory workout is taught by a certified, experienced trainer who coaches you, and that makes a difference. No one wants to go into Push or All Out on their own. Orangetheory trainers do more than just teach; they inspire. They create energy. They educate in a mass format. They create an environment, a community where people feel welcomed. When you exercise in a group, an amazing team dynamic starts to happen. It's one reason lifelong friendships happen in group workouts, and we see the same thing at Orangetheory.

- **Proper form.** As I said earlier, fitness is about learning physical skills. Your Orangetheory trainer teaches you the proper way to execute each movement, whether you're using the water rower or performing a dumbbell fly. Our trainers each go through a rigorous training program to ensure that they know how to coach, demonstrate proper form, inspire, motivate, and make sure that you have fun!

- **Constant change, constant challenge.** Colonel Sanders used to say it was his secret sauce in the batter of his fried chicken that made it so delicious. Well, I took the science of metabolically training the body—and my own background and experience—to create *our* secret sauce. What's in the secret sauce? The way our training blocks (specific sections of the workout) are built, how our ESP formula is used, and our systematic approach to the design of the workouts. Now my team of Orangetheory exercise experts design 30 different workouts a month to constantly challenge the body in different ways, which means **you do a different workout every day.**

- **Cutting-edge technology.** Our proprietary heart rate–monitoring devices and software let you check your heart rate and adjust your intensity depending on your goals. That immediate, real-time feedback tells you that not only is your workout going to create results—but also it's doing so already.

- **Success breeds success.** The best workout in the world won't make a difference if people won't do it. I wanted people to finish a workout feeling like "I did this, and I can do it again." (In fact, **I often talk about turning "I can't" into "I can."**) I had to make sure people would want to come back, and that meant people had to enjoy it! Even though there's discomfort, people leave the Orangetheory studio feeling accomplished—and that feeling bleeds over into

15

other areas of their lives. They learn how to **get comfortable being uncomfortable**, and mastering that empowers them.

Orangetheory: The Answer

So what is Orangetheory, in short? It's your workout staple. It's that multivitamin you take two or three times a week to **metabolically charge the body**—to have more energy, to lose weight, to feel great, and simply **to become the best physical version of you**.

Chances are you own a cell phone (that you probably never leave home without). When it starts to run out of power, you plug it into your charger. That's what you do at Orangetheory. **Your body is the phone, and the workout is the charger**. The workout gives you the metabolically charged body (Sick of that phrase yet? You'll hear it lots more!) that changes everything. It changes how you look. It changes how you feel. It changes how you live.

So how I did come up with it? Read on for the rest of the story.

2

A New Approach:
How Orangetheory
was Created

My interest in fitness pretty much started at birth. One of my earliest memories was watching Jack LaLanne on TV. He captivated me! I loved that one-piece jumpsuit that never had a wrinkle it in. While all of the other kids would want to watch other shows, I would be watching Jack and all of his strange exercises. I'd stand in our living room while watching the black-and-white television and mimicking all of his moves.

I grew up loving the feeling of being active. But that was before Title IV and before many sports options were available for girls. Cheerleading was as athletic as I could get, and I was a pretty awesome cheerleader! I also swam and biked whenever I could and ice-skated during the winters.

I owe my love of being physical to my father, Arthur Calandrelli. He was a standout football player in high school and was offered a punting position with the Toronto Argonauts in the 1940s. Instead, he accepted the full football scholarship he was offered from Canisius College in Buffalo, New York, so he could get a college degree. He was the only one in his Italian immigrant family of eight brothers and sisters to go to college.

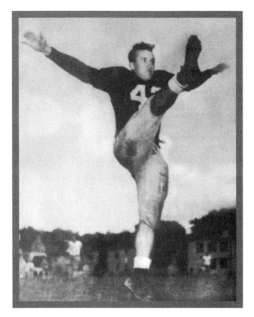

My dad, Arthur Calandrelli, as a college punter.

In college, he punted an average of 47.5 yards—and held the national college punting record for 12 years!

After college, my dad married my mom, Rose Maglio, and they had four kids: Arthur Junior, me, Cindy, and Chris. My dad became a phys ed teacher, and all the kids in the neighborhood would gather to play in our front yard. He'd lead games of kickball, kick the can, you name it. I remember that all of our neighbors' yards were green and gorgeous while ours looked like a dirt pit from all the kids playing there! No one else wanted their kids running around on their lawns, but my father loved it. He was a very physical person and loved teaching high school phys ed for decades. His last coaching job was at Niagara Falls High School; after that, he took a job with the board of education. He was so well known around town that everyone simply called him "Coach."

Coach was one of those teachers who went *beyond*. He always knew he wanted to be a teacher. He cared about his students, especially his football players. He spent long afternoons and evenings coaching the football team. His school was one of the poorer ones in the district, and I remember the players' uniforms often had holes. Some of his players didn't have a lot of support at home or had families who were struggling. That just made my dad work harder, and my mother always supported him. When we were little, my mother would bring us to the park where he coached his team nearly every night. She would feed us dinner at home, and then we'd drive over to the park and sit on the sidelines and watch him work with his players.

A lot of what I heard and saw in terms of how he interacted with his players really made an impression on me. I saw he built his players up. He never tore them down; he taught them to believe in themselves and "momentum shift" up, helping them focus on what they had instead of what they didn't have. I remember him talking to my mother one night about one of his players, Ernest, who was a high school running back. Ernest didn't have a great home environment and was starting to get in trouble on the streets.

My dad encouraged Ernest to commit to staying out of trouble and to focus on football and school. Ernest had speed and size, and my dad told him he'd help him get a football scholarship so he could go to college. Years later, at my dad's funeral, Ernest stood in line with many other mourners to pay their respects. He grabbed my hand and said, "Ellen, your father kept me out of jail. Thanks to him, I got into college and graduated, and now I have a great job and three kids. He always made me believe in myself when I didn't."

That was my dad! He was a master at helping his players momentum shift up. That's how he lived his whole life—focusing on what he had, not on what he didn't. In 1966, his football team, the Niagara Falls Wildcats, was named one of the three best teams in New York State and second in the *country* for defensive points allowed, with a total of only 20 points for the entire season! This was a huge accomplishment. Many of his players that year received full college scholarships, something that never would have happened without his coaching.

Those evenings spent watching him coach his team—both at practices and at games—made me who I am. (So, thank you, Dad.)

But I wasn't sure that I wanted to commit to a career in fitness until I was in high school. I was an A student, and my parents, especially my dad, really wanted me to go to college. They expected it. By my senior year, all of my friends were deciding what they wanted to be and talking about their college and career plans. Everyone seemed to be going into business and other lucrative careers, but that didn't appeal to me.

I remember sitting down in my living room with my father in our modest three-bedroom house in Niagara Falls. This was the mid-'70s, and it wasn't the time to be a teacher—there were already about five million teachers, so it wasn't a field to go into if you wanted a job.

My dad asked, "What do you think you'd love doing for many, many years?"

"I want to do what *you* do," I told him. "I want to be a phys ed teacher. But I don't know whether I'd be able to get a job."

I'll never forget what he said next: "Don't worry about that. Whenever you do something you're passionate about, you'll always find work. And you'll always be great at it." That conversation—and his faith in me—was really the beginning of my fitness career!

My Entry into the Fitness Field

The summer before college, when I was 17, I got my first job. My first employer was the YWCA in Niagara Falls, New York. My job was to strap my women members into these "fat-jiggle" machines. I'd strap them in, set the timer for 15 minutes, and then unstrap them and send them on their way. I guess you would call me a personal trainer and the fat-jiggle machines the fitness technology of the 1970s.

In addition to the jiggle machines, the YWCA also had a wooden fat-roller machine. You'd sit on it and roll your hips and thighs over it. The idea was that it was supposed to roll your fat away, like a rolling pin rolls away air bubbles from dough. Women were told it would fix their cellulite problem. (Hmmm, yeah, that darn cellulite! We're still trying to find a solution for it.)

These machines were about instant gratification. People may have believed that they were doing something, but nothing changed. What I did learn early on, though, was that people want the quickest results in the shortest period of time. That lesson would actually be instrumental decades later when I created my Ultimate Workout, which would become Orangetheory.

Fitness over the Decades

The '60s: Bodybuilding and Free Weights

When I started working in the fitness industry, bodybuilding and free weights were still very popular. People such as Vic Tanny, who pioneered the first version of a health club, and Joe Weider, considered the father of bodybuilding by many, brought attention to the sport. Weider opened his first Gold's Gym in 1965, and the most visible bodybuilder, Arnold Schwarzenegger, amazed the public with his eye-popping muscles.

Guys started going crazy for free weights. The weight room became a more popular place for both bodybuilders and everyday exercisers at gyms throughout the country, and more people starting joining health clubs.

The '70s: Kenneth Cooper and Aerobics

In the '70s, bodybuilding was still popular, but by the time I was working as a teen helping women jiggle away their fat, the fitness craze was well under way. In the '70s, the buzzword in fitness was "aerobics." Fitness pioneer Dr. Kenneth Cooper introduced the concept of aerobics and helped start get America exercising. Author Jim Fixx helped create the running boom, and suddenly millions of people started lacing up their shoes and hitting the streets. The popularity of road races such as 5Ks, 10Ks, and even marathons exploded.

Inside the gym, things were just as exciting. In 1976, I started teaching dance aerobics. That's what people wanted. People such as Jacki Sorensen, who invented the concept of combining dance and aerobics, made an impact. Sorensen took this whole concept of aerobic conditioning and blended it with dance, and women loved it. I loved it, too. I loved learning the routines and then freestyling, or creating my own choreography, too. I knew at this time that large-group training was for me.

The YMCA I worked at had a strength-training room, a cardio room with treadmills and stationary bicycles, and an aerobic room. I spent most of my time in the aerobic room, where I taught and took classes. I loved the energy of group exercise classes. But one day I decided to venture into the strength-training room. Every single man there (and there were only men in there in those days) stopped what he was doing to stare at me. My heart rate was in the Orange Zone just standing still!

Thank goodness a member who knew me well came up to me and showed me how to use the strength machines. I loved the new challenge. I spent three days a week in that room, and eventually the guys got used to me. I even started bringing a few of the brave females who took my aerobics class in there to strength train and started to recognize how effective weights were in terms of building a lean, sculpted body.

The '80s: Personal Training

In the '80s, personal training really started to take off at the fitness facilities with which I was associated. People were busy and did not really know the best way to use the weight machines, dumbbells, and cardio equipment in the gym (and still don't). Personal trainers became the answer. But it wasn't until around the end of the decade that this unregulated fitness boom—as far as this new definition of a personal fitness trainer—became somewhat regulated.

The American College of Sports Medicine was the first fitness organization to offer certifications for personal trainers to help ensure that trainers were qualified; it started certifying personal trainers in 1975. Other fitness organizations started offering certification programs as well, and personal trainers began to become a regular sight on health club floors.

However, group fitness continued to be popular in the '80s as well. Dance aerobics classes continued to attract millions of women, and the end of the '80s, step aerobics, initially created by fitness pro Gin Miller, started the stepping craze.

The '90s: Mind-Body Fitness

The '90s brought a new spin to group fitness with the introduction of Spinning, a group cycling class. Other group classes such as Tae Bo and kickboxing attracted new members to the gym.

We also started to see an increased interest in mind-body workouts such as Pilates and yoga. By the mid-'90s, numerous celebrities were crediting their lean shapes to Pilates, and the general public followed suit. People were starting to realize that there was more to exercise than the physical; engaging the brain was as important as engaging the body.

The '00s until Now: Niche Programming

The renewed interest in group classes led to an explosion in health clubs around the turn of the twenty-first century. Commercial fitness facilities were cropping up everywhere, and other facilities, such as country clubs, private clubs, and hotels, jumped aboard. Suddenly, you could find a gym or workout facility on just about every corner.

Since 2000, we've seen the continued popularity of both personal trainers and group exercise classes. What's new, however, is what we call niche fitness; it has gained a strong foothold. While some fitness trends are fading (think Tae Bo and Jazzercise), plenty of new facilities are devoted to specific workouts: think CrossFit, Ballet Barre, yoga studios, and boxing clubs. In fact, in 2013, niche, or boutique, fitness facilities represented 21 percent of all clubs, according to the International Health, Racquet & Sportsclub Association.

Orangetheory technically falls into that category of niche fitness. However, there's a big difference. I still have a Pilates studio, and I personally love to do Pilates, but Pilates can't do it all. Pilates' primary focus is on strengthening your inside muscles. Think of it as your vitamin A for the day.

But Pilates—and other workouts that target one specific area of fitness—are only one type of vitamin. To be the best you that you can be, **you still need a multivitamin to metabolically charge the body**. That's Orangetheory.

The Story of Orangetheory

Because I'd been in the fitness industry for decades, I had lived through all of these changes. I had firsthand experience in teaching different types of classes and using different training methods with members of both genders and of all ages. I'd seen plenty of fitness trends come and go. But my initial intention never was to create my own workout.

I started on this entrepreneurial journey (a journey I didn't even know I was on!) after I was let go from what I thought at the time was my dream job. In 1993, I was hired as the director at a high-end private spa and fitness facility in Miami. In addition to managing the spa, I taught group fitness classes.

While there, I quickly created an identity as a recognized fitness professional in the community. I was on television three times a week on the local Fox affiliate and offered viewers fitness tips. I wrote Q&A fitness columns for *The Miami Herald*. I was often quoted in magazines, newspapers, and other media as a fitness expert. I judged area fitness contests and hosted fashion shows. I even sold fitness equipment such as heart rate monitors and home gym equipment on QVC, the shopping network! I was considered *the* go-to fitness expert in Miami at the time.

Well, none of that mattered when my boss called me into his office. He told me he was letting me go.

I was devastated. Suddenly, it didn't matter that I was the local fitness expert. Now I was just a 40-year-old single parent with a nine-year-old son and no job. That's when I thought of my dad and about momentum shifting, of focusing on what you have instead of what you don't have. So, when I could have climbed under the covers with a pint of Häagen-Dazs, I instead pushed ahead. I couldn't afford to crawl under the covers, both literally and figuratively!

I thought about what I had, and what I had was a lot of experience teaching group exercise classes. I knew I was a great instructor. In fact, I was already involved with a small Spinning program at a Gold's Gym near my house. The classes were popular, but the pay was nowhere enough to support myself and my son.

I also had a Pilates certification, so I started doing one-on-one Pilates classes out of my house. I was paid more for these classes than at the gym, and I soon got so busy I was taking two clients on the hour. Some days I would have two women pulling in my driveway and two women pulling out of my driveway, every hour, on the hour, from 6:00 a.m. to 9:00 p.m.! (I still have no idea what kind of business the neighbors thought I had going on!)

Over about a year and a half, I continued to build momentum, and I ended up borrowing some money to open the first Pilates studio in Fort Lauderdale. This was when I first started to use my own creative design in a group class format. I had 12 Pilates machines, so I used the principles of Pilates and my own fitness knowledge and background to create my own class, called Pilates-Fit.

After a few years of doing this, I noticed my clients were frustrated with the fact that Pilates gave them sculpted, strong muscles—but that those muscles were buried under a few layers of fat. Pilates is not a high-metabolic, or fat-burning, workout. Many of my clients were going to personal trainers in addition to doing Pilates. Most of the trainers had them weight train and do the treadmill for 15 to 30 minutes before their session; others tried Spinning or jogging on their own, but almost no one saw the results they were looking for.

They didn't have a program of structure to follow. They didn't know how much cardio to do, or how hard, or for how long. They didn't know how to strength train. Their efforts, no matter what they were doing, weren't being monitored. So I decided to create what I would call the Ultimate Workout. I found a space three times the size of my Pilates studio—and three times the rent—and signed a lease. I would move in within six months. (In chapters 5–7, you'll learn more about how I made this transition and the lessons I learned from it—and how they can apply to your life as well.)

I couldn't find that perfect metabolic workout that included and addressed all aspects of fitness, so I decided to create my own. Given my years of experience, I decided the perfect metabolic workout needed to feature the following:

- **A program performed in a group environment.** Group fitness has always been my exercise of choice. The first five minutes of most cardio workouts are miserable. Your muscles are waking up; it's becoming harder to breathe. You're just starting to feel some discomfort. When you're in a group, you're not concentrating on that; you're more energized because you're with other people. You're distracted—in a good way—and have less of a chance to start complaining to yourself or to turn the "I can't" channel on. (More about "I can't" versus "I can" later.) I've seen that members are more accountable when they work out in a group. They work harder. They push themselves more. Then there are always people in the group who are having an amazing day, and if you're not having one, you can pull off of their energy. Groups have social benefits as well. You build relationships with each other. Sometimes you see the same person during your workouts more than you see members of your own family! You bond. I've witnessed lifelong friendships from group classes. Another reason for group exercise is that people love the energetic atmosphere. People want to leave their dreaded day spent in a cubicle—and the people or things stressing them out—behind. They want to escape into great music and inspiring coaching, and I knew that had to be a component of my Ultimate Workout.

- **A program that was based on science.** My workout had to be based on the science of the body, on physiology. I didn't want to create some fad exercise concept; I wanted something that would produce results, based on my understanding of the science of training the body from both my educational background and real-life results in the gym. I used decades' worth of research to create a workout that would burn fat and build muscle.

- **A program that made people feel successful.** I knew that my workout had to be physiologically sound, but it had to be psychologically and behaviorally sound as well. When it comes to the psychology of exercise, it's pretty simple. I knew that people would need to feel successful to continue coming back. **The best exercise program in the world is useless if people won't do it**. I knew that I needed my members to feel successful, to never feel "less than." That's why I used the word "options" instead of "modifications." Sure, you can offer modifications to members. That's what we're trained to do as group exercise instructors. But I found that my members didn't feel successful when they had to modify a move. They felt conspicuous. They felt weak. They felt less than. Well, an option is different. An option doesn't have that same connotation. My goal was for everyone to feel successful both during the workout and afterward. I created the categories of Walkers/Joggers/Runners so that no one would feel left out. My language choices and programming were designed to make everyone feel like a success.

- **A program that engaged people.** I knew that I had to create a design that would engage people and make them *want* to come back. Part of that was helping them feel successful. But I also had to figure out a way to encourage members to push themselves beyond what they would normally do. They were going to have to feel uncomfortable, at least for short periods of time. I had to help them

learn how to be comfortable being uncomfortable. The program I created would have to be so engaging that members would never look at the clock. I'd have to create enough variety and challenges that the hour-long workout would feel like it was flying by!

- **A program that required only three sessions a week.** Lack of time is the number one reason given for not exercising. That is why I wanted to create a workout that members would have to do only three times a week. Almost all people can make that kind of commitment, especially when they know they're going to see a change in their bodies, their mental outlooks, and their lives.

- **A program that was the right intensity.** As I said above, I knew that people had to be willing to push themselves above and beyond what they would normally do. I didn't want a program that would let people undertrain, but I also didn't want people to overtrain! I had to develop a program that would enable people to reach the appropriate intensities for the appropriate amount of time. That's why I used the five-zone heart rate system to create the workout.

Testing the Workout

Now that I had these six factors in mind, I had six months to get the workout nailed down. Another nonnegotiable for me was to be very consistent with piloting the workout. I put a class on my Pilates schedule that I called the Ultimate Workout and did it outside with my members. I didn't have a room that was designed to hold the class, nor did I have all of the equipment I'd wind up using, such as the rower.

So, six days a week I would take whoever would sign up and run them from stop sign to stop sign at different intensities—Base, Push, and All Out. I gave them each a weight bar (I didn't have room for a dumbbell supply) and a BOSU, a balance trainer that stands for "both sides up," and we'd train in the parking lot. I had to be very persistent. When it just did not feel right or I would get input from my members that made sense, I would make slight changes and then do it again, and again, and again.

A huge external sense of urgency existed during this time. Recall that I had six months before I opened my new, larger, much more expensive studio and it would be showtime! This was a huge motivator. Today, I often use what I call "internal self-imposed urgency" in my business (more about that in later chapters).

Initially, we were using perceived exertion to track workout intensity. There are different ways to measure perceived exertion, but I had my members use a simple 1–10 scale:

- 1   No activity

- 2–3   Light activity

- 4–6   Moderate activity (Base, or challenging but doable)

- 7–8   Heavy activity (Push, or uncomfortable)

- 9–10   Very heavy activity (All Out, or very uncomfortable)

In addition to the interval training and strength training, I knew I wanted to include power moves. I had members doing explosive plyometric, or jumping, moves, but they didn't like it, and I knew I was putting them at risk for injury. I had to figure out a way to include power in the workout. That's when I heard about Josh Crosby, a national championship rower, who was teaching rowing classes in California. I called him out of the blue and told him I wanted to meet him.

I think he thought I was crazy, but I flew to California the next week to take some of his classes and learn more about rowing and how it could fit into my Ultimate Workout program. (Crosby is now part of Orangetheory's Fitness Advisory Board.) Rowing gave me the power aspect of the workout my members needed, providing full-body power and strength with zero impact.

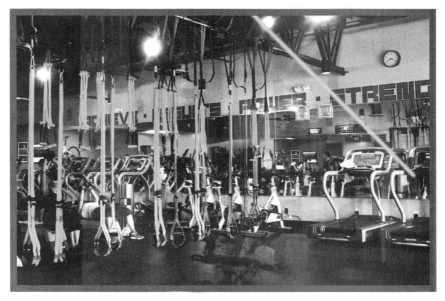

The TRX straps I started using at Ellen's.

I still needed to tweak the program, though. While I was running people around the parking lot, I knew I wanted the workout to include intervals and weight training that would create muscle overload. The missing link was what I call the inside muscles, the muscles that Pilates does such a good job of targeting. In 2001, a Navy SEAL named Randy Hetrick created TRX straps, canvas straps that attach to a wall and let you strength train using your body weight. I knew TRX straps would be a great way to train those inside foundational muscles, especially for my members who weren't doing Pilates or yoga on a regular basis.

I had my members perform the workout dozens of times over the next six months, continually tweaking and modifying the Ultimate Workout. How did I do it? First, I had that external drive—the lease on my new studio, which was three times more expensive than my current studio, was going to start on April 1, 2007, whether I was ready or not! This was definitely a Push for me, and I used the power of relentless focus (more about that in chapter 6) to drive myself harder than I ever had before.

Just one week before my new studio, Ellen's, opened, the equipment was delivered. Finally, I chose music for the workout—I knew from my experience teaching literally thousands of classes that the right music would make a huge difference for my members. For the Ultimate Workout, I chose music with a typical tempo of 125–145 BPM, or beats per minute. Research has shown that music is a powerful motivator, reduces perceived exertion, and improves exercise adherence, even when you're exercising at a high intensity.

I had the studio. I had the equipment. I had the workout. I had the music. It was showtime! The first day of operation, I had nearly 100 classes running, including 35 Ultimate Workout classes! At the time, I had no idea that just three years later, I'd be franchising my workout and that people would do more than a million Orangetheory workouts each month!

From the Ultimate Workout to Orangetheory

Even after I launched the Ultimate Workout, fine-tuning was still involved. I continued to experiment with different formats, musical choices, and exercise moves.

In 2010, the Ultimate Workout was rebranded as the Orangetheory Fitness workout. "Orange" stands for physical energy, stimulation, and rejuvenation. "Theory" stands for getting the heart rate over 84 percent (hitting the Orange, and sometimes Red, Zone) for 12–20 minutes during each hour-long workout.

Since I franchised the Ultimate Workout to become Orangetheory, we have continued to tweak and modify the Orangetheory workouts. About three years ago, we developed the ESP program, which stands for Endurance/Strength/Power. Besides offering a total-body workout, each day's workout has a specific emphasis. Members are kept psychologically as well as physically challenged in meeting each day's goals.

ESP keeps members stimulated, interested, and engaged. Every day is different, and every workout is different. That's part of the secret sauce of how we design the workouts to change every day and send the workouts to the studios. Our trainers also go through rigorous training to ensure that they understand how to coach, motivate, and lead our members. So if a new member's form isn't quite right when performing a dip, an Orangetheory trainer will show the member an option (not a modification) so that he or she can feel successful. Each trainer is there to ensure that every member gets a great workout—and will want to come back!

At Orangetheory, we began using heart rate monitors, using our own OTbeat-branded technology. OTbeat is available only in Orangetheory studios and lets our members track their intensity throughout the workout so they do not train too hard or not hard enough. Splat Points and heart rate information give members real-time information about whether they need to pick it up or back off a little during their workouts.

The Fitness Multivitamin

I want to be clear that while I love Orangetheory, I understand that everyone is different. Different people like to do different workouts and for different reasons. So I still maintain a studio (the original Ellen's in Fort Lauderdale) that includes a Ballet Barre studio, a hot yoga studio, a Pilates studio, and a small Spinning studio. Members love these classes! But Orangetheory is the multivitamin workout where you will get everything you need to stimulate metabolism at the highest level, live in your best body, and feel like you're the best *you*.

That's why I do Orangetheory even today. My Pilates workout is my vitamin A and my yoga my vitamin B, but Orangetheory is my multivitamin—everything I need.

So what am I saying? Continue to go to yoga. Go to CrossFit. Play tennis. Run or walk. But two or three times a week, take your multivitamin, Orangetheory.

From the Ultimate Workout to Orangetheory

I did not set out to be the creator of a workout that has been performed more than 14 million times since Orangetheory was created. All I did was follow my passion. I wanted to have a successful, boutique-style studio where I could use my talents to help other people, and, today, Orangetheory is the result. The best part is that we at Orangetheory continue to adapt, to change, and to grow—and to help our franchisees and our members do the same.

Continually challenging the body is the key to a metabolically charged body. Continually challenging ourselves is our mission at Orangetheory. Being the best version of me is my goal for myself. That's the goal for all of us at Orangetheory as well—from the management team, to the corporate staff, to the fitness team, to the franchisees, to the trainers. We're all trying to be the best version of ourselves that we can be, and Orangetheory helps us do that.

Now that you know how Orangetheory was created and developed, let's delve into the science behind what makes it so successful.

The Science behind Orangetheory: Why the Workout Works

Last chapter you learned how—and why—I created the Ultimate Workout, which became Orangetheory. In this chapter, I'll show you why this program is so effective at creating a metabolically charged body.

Let's start with looking at the three sciences behind the workout: physiology, psychology, and behavioral science.

Physiology: The Science of the Body and How It Works

As you saw in the preceding chapters, the four basic elements of the Orangetheory hour-long workout are:

- Cardiovascular interval training.

- Strength training for outside muscles.

- Strengthening inside muscles.

- Power training.

I chose these specific elements after decades of working in the fitness industry and learning as much as I could about how the body works and responds to exercise. Let's start by looking at the physiology behind the Orangetheory workout.

Cardiovascular exercise is at the heart (pardon the pun) of any workout. The benefits of regular cardio exercise include:

- A stronger, healthier heart and lungs.

- Reduced risk of developing heart disease and high blood pressure.

- Reduced risk of developing metabolic syndrome and diabetes.

- Improved muscular and bone strength.

- Improved ability to lose weight and maintain a healthy body weight.

- Reduction in depression and anxiety.

- Improved cognitive function.

- Improved overall life expectancy.

- Improved mood.

However, not all cardio exercise is created equal. What I've found is that people do too much cardio (often at the exclusion of other things, such as strength training). Or they do too little. Or they exercise too hard—or not hard enough! When you do any of these things, you compromise your body's response to the exercise, and **you reduce the benefits you receive from it**.

Interval Training: The Secret to a Metabolically Charged Body

So what's the answer? Interval training. Interval training has been around since the early twentieth century, when runners started using intervals as part of their training regimes. Competitive runners found that incorporating higher-intensity intervals, or amounts of time, during their regular workouts made for faster race times. This was a novel approach; until then, the thinking had been that the more miles, the better. Run more miles and you'd drop your race times.

Finding that the opposite was true—that runners could run less mileage (but occasionally at faster paces) and produce faster race times—was the beginning of a dramatic change in cardio training for coaches, athletes, fitness professionals, and everyday athletes alike.

However, interval training does much more than help runners go faster. Decades of research have found that interval training is superior to other types of cardio training, such as steady state, where you exercise at a consistent, doable pace. Interval training changes your body literally from the inside out. Let's look at what's happening in the body when you're interval training.

You create an EPOC response.

Remember EPOC is short for excess postexercise oxygen consumption. That fancy phrase simply means that your body revs its metabolism so high during the workout that you continue to burn extra calories (think of splatting those fat cells) for up to 24–36 hours after your workout.

High-intensity interval training is proven to create EPOC, or afterburn. The afterburn comes from the fact that the body has to work harder at the mitochondrial level to build those oxygen stores back up to restore all of the body's energetic systems.

Sometimes when I teach a class, I'll make a comment such as, "Let's blow up those mitochondria!" If you remember the sidebar from chapter 1, mitochondria are the power plants of your body's cells. Inside all of your body's cells are tiny furnaces, the mitochondria. The mitochondria use primarily sugar, or glucose, and fat to power the cell and create ATP, or adenosine triphosphate. That ATP is cellular energy.

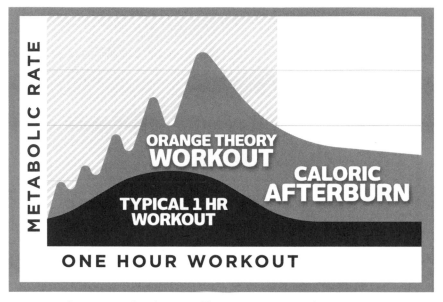

Orangetheory's afterburn effect means you burn more calories for hours post-workout.

Just as a furnace must have oxygen to work, your cells require oxygen to burn and create energy. The more oxygen, the higher the flame, so to speak, and the volume and density of the mitochondria increase. The result is **more ATP = more energy for you**, not only during your workout but also for the rest of your day!

When your body's cardio system and muscles are overloaded, as in Push and All Out, more oxygen is delivered to the mitochondria (remember the taxicabs?) to create more ATP, the energy for your body's cells. That process, called mitochondrial biogenesis, was described more than 40 years ago by Washington University Professor John Holloszy, of St. Louis, Missouri. This process basically means that mitochondria in the cell build volume and become denser in response to increased demand during higher intensities. There is also an increase in a concentration of what is called cytochrome c, which is found in the inner membrane of the mitochondria and is crucial for aerobic energy production.

You increase your VO$_2$ max.

As your body's mitochondria become denser and larger, your body's VO$_2$ max increases. VO$_2$ max is a marker of how efficiently your body uses oxygen. It generally is the highest in very fit athletes and drops gradually over time due to aging. However, training your body with Pushes and All Outs can increase your VO$_2$ max regardless of age.

Chances are that unless you're a trained athlete, you don't know what your VO$_2$ max is. You probably don't even care. However, a simple way to track your fitness levels is to take your heart rate upon awakening in the morning. Your resting heart rate—the number of beats per minute—is another indicator of how fit and healthy your cardiovascular system is. After a month or two of training at Orangetheory, you'll see that number start to drop.

You'll also notice that you have to walk, jog, run, or row faster to get into the Green, Orange, or Red Zone. Thanks to the increase in mitochondria

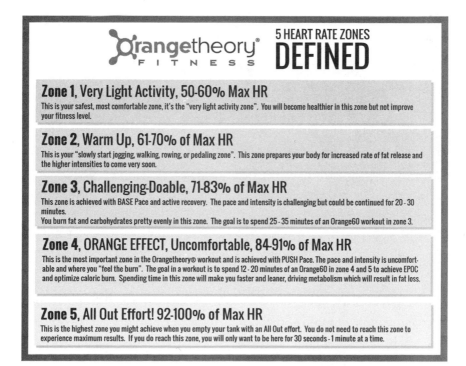

Orangetheory® FITNESS
5 HEART RATE ZONES DEFINED

Zone 1, Very Light Activity, 50-60% Max HR
This is your safest, most comfortable zone, it's the "very light activity zone". You will become healthier in this zone but not improve your fitness level.

Zone 2, Warm Up, 61-70% of Max HR
This is your "slowly start jogging, walking, rowing, or pedaling zone". This zone prepares your body for increased rate of fat release and the higher intensities to come very soon.

Zone 3, Challenging-Doable, 71-83% of Max HR
This zone is achieved with BASE Pace and active recovery. The pace and intensity is challenging but could be continued for 20 - 30 minutes.
You burn fat and carbohydrates pretty evenly in this zone. The goal is to spend 25 - 35 minutes of an Orange60 workout in zone 3.

Zone 4, ORANGE EFFECT, Uncomfortable, 84-91% of Max HR
This is the most important zone in the Orangetheory® workout and is achieved with PUSH Pace. The pace and intensity is uncomfortable and where you "feel the burn". The goal in a workout is to spend 12 - 20 minutes of an Orange60 in zone 4 and 5 to achieve EPOC and optimize caloric burn. Spending time in this zone will make you faster and leaner, driving metabolism which will result in fat loss.

Zone 5, All Out Effort! 92-100% of Max HR
This is the highest zone you might achieve when you empty your tank with an All Out effort. You do not need to reach this zone to experience maximum results. If you do reach this zone, you will only want to be here for 30 seconds - 1 minute at a time.

and the increased volume of oxygen, your VO$_2$ max is now higher—and what may have really challenged you before just doesn't seem that hard anymore!

You use all three muscle fiber types.

Besides creating larger, stronger mitochondria, which produce more ATP, interval training uses all three types of muscle fibers.

The three basic types of muscle fibers are:

- Type I, or slow-twitch, muscle fibers.

- Type IIa, or fast-twitch oxidative, fibers.

- Type IIb, or fast-twitch glycolic, fibers.

Each type of muscle fiber has different abilities. Type I fibers have high endurance but low force/power/speed production. Type IIb have low endurance but high force/power/speed production. Type IIa fall in between the two; they have less endurance than type I but more endurance than type IIb and more force/power/speed production than type I and less force/power/speed production than type IIb.

Each of us is genetically predisposed to have more of certain muscle fiber types and less of others. So an athlete with a higher proportion of type I fibers would be more likely to excel at endurance events such as marathons (thanks to his or her slow-twitch muscles), while an athlete with more type IIb would be better at sprinting. Unfortunately, you can't get more of any of the different muscle types. However, you can train them to improve their function.

The interval training that Orangetheory workouts are designed around is designed to recruit and train all three different muscle types. In the Green Zone, you're using mostly type I fibers, which improve endurance. In the Orange Zone, you're using more type IIa fast twitch, which help improve force and power, and in the Red Zone, you're using those type IIb muscles that generate the most force and power.

Steady-state or lower-intensity workouts target mostly type I muscles, because you're not pushing yourself hard enough to have to recruit type IIa and type IIb muscles. That's a problem. First, if you never use those muscle fibers, you're using less muscle overall, which means you burn fewer calories. Second, if you never use your fast-twitch muscles, they shrink and lose their size and strength. You become weaker and less able to generate the kind of force and power you need to sprint or jump or exercise at high intensity.

As I already said, when you train in the Green, Orange, and Red Zones, you'll use all three types of fibers during your Orangetheory interval workouts.

The strength training you do at Orangetheory is designed to train all three fiber types as well. When you do sets with a weight that's heavy enough that you can lift it only five to 10 times with good form, you're training your fast-twitch muscles and adding lean muscle to your body. When you do a set with a weight that you can lift for 12 reps or more, you're training more slow-twitch muscles and creating more muscular endurance. And when you do a set of eight to 12 reps, you're training those type IIa muscles, the in-between muscles.

That's a lot of talk about muscle fibers, but all you need to know is that the Orangetheory interval training and weight training target and train all three types. Training the fast-twitch muscles (IIa and IIb) is especially important for a lean, healthy body. In one study conducted at the State University of New York at Syracuse, researchers found that training fast-twitch fibers by running at a very high intensity for 10 minutes *tripled* cytochrome c concentration, which you'll recall is essential for energy production.

So what do you need to know about the three types of muscle fibers? In short, it's pretty simple: **the more muscle fibers you use, total, the more calories you burn**. And the more muscle you have, the better. In addition to burning more calories, having more muscle:

- Makes you stronger.

- Increases the strength of your bones and joints.

- Improves immune function.

- Improves your balance.

- Improves sleep.

- Reduces symptoms of some conditions such as arthritis.

- Reduces depression.

- Improves mood and self-esteem.

You combat the natural aging process.

Another important aspect of interval training is that studies suggest it can delay the chromosomal damage that occurs when we age. You probably already know that our chromosomes are made up of strands of DNA (deoxyribonucleic acid), which contains our genetic material. At the tip of each chromosomal strand are telomeres, which protect our DNA, kind of like the way the plastic tip of a shoelace keeps it from unraveling. Well, as we age, those telomeres get shorter and offer less protection to our DNA. Over time, that can lead to the death of the DNA cells, which can in turn lead to diseases such as cancer.

Scary stuff, huh? Well, a study in the *Journal of Mechanisms of Aging and Development* from 2010 suggests that interval training can help prevent telomere shortening as we age, in turn protecting your body's DNA. Other, newer research supports this idea. This means that interval training *may* play a role in protecting you from seeing as many age-related changes (think wrinkles and fine lines) as you get older and may make you less susceptible to serious diseases such as cancer.

You produce more human growth hormone.

Human growth hormone, or HGH, is a hormone that stimulates cell growth and reproduction. As you get older, though, your body naturally produces less of this HGH. That's probably why a 41-year-old friend of mine, Debbie, just told me she's been getting HGH shots!

Well, forget the shots. A study in the 2003 *Journal of Sports Medicine* found that staying above lactate threshold for at least 10 minutes elicits the secretion of HGH. Our Orangetheory formula of getting 12–20 Splat Points is the equivalent of staying in the lactate threshold for 12–20 minutes and will help ensure that your body produces more of this essential hormone. After I told Debbie about this, she ditched the HGH shots—in favor of Orangetheory three times a week!

You build your brain.

Studies published in the past year show that very high-intensity intervals or sprints (our All Outs) increase the formation of something called BDNF, or brain-derived neurotropic factor. BDNF is used by the brain to aid memory, learning, and reasoning.

What this means is that doing All Outs basically lets you create new brain cells, which can assist with better mid- and long-term memory. It may even help make you smarter. Whether you're a college student shooting for straight As, a business owner with a lot of balls in the air, a mom who has to manage her own life and that of her family, or a baby boomer, this is good news! (Hey, I'm a baby boomer looking for every advantage I can get, as I want to thrive in my body for as long as possible. And if Orangetheory helps me find my keys in the morning, that's a win!)

You reduce your body fat.

Weight loss is the goal of many Orangetheory members, and research shows that interval training reduces body fat more effectively than steady-state cardio. It's also more effective than steady state at reducing abdominal fat.

Other studies have proven that interval training helps your body burn more stored body fat, which also helps you achieve the sculpted, lean look you're pursuing.

Strength Training: The Key to a Leaner, Fitter Body

Interval training is at the heart of the Orangetheory workout. However, three other aspects of the program help make it so successful. Those are strength training for the outside muscles, strengthening the inside muscles, and rowing, which I'll discuss in a bit.

I already explained the importance of training all three types of muscle fibers in the above section on interval training, but let me just touch again on the importance of creating and maintaining lean muscle. Orangetheory's interval training and its ESP (Endurance/Strength/Power) routines put muscle on the human body in a manageable, systematic way with a metabolic emphasis.

It's also important to note that the program targets both the outside, or mover, muscles and the inside, or stabilizer, muscles. Orangetheory is designed to create an equal level of strength in both muscle areas. Over the years, I've observed many muscle imbalances in members that prevented them from getting ideal results—and resulted in a lot of aches, pains, and sometimes injuries. That's why you work both kinds of muscles in every class.

Outside Muscles (Your Movers)

I sometimes call the outside muscles your "mirror muscles," or your moving muscles, because they're the muscles that *move* your body. Your inside muscles *stabilize* your body.

To train your outside muscles, we use a variety of strength-training equipment at Orangetheory: free weights; BOSUs; benches; and ab dollies, little scooters to help target your core as well as functional body weight movements.

To create (and maintain) muscle tissue, you must progressively overload it by gradually increasing the amount of stress you put on it during exercise.

Research has shown that to do this, you challenge muscles by changing the volume, intensity, and frequency of training. Orangetheory uses the ESP approach, which varies each of these three factors depending on the day to avoid over- or undertraining any particular muscle group. That means you're building muscle, not losing it—and your body burns more calories maintaining muscle than maintaining fat.

Inside Muscles (Your Stabilizers)

These are deep muscles hidden under and behind your movement muscles. The TRX straps used in Orangetheory improve strength in the three primary areas of stabilization that make up the foundation of your body:

- The trunk. These are your deep abdominals (transverse abdominus, mulitfidus, and internal and external oblique muscles).

- Shoulder stabilization (scapula). These inside muscles include the lower trapezius, serratus anterior, and rhomboids.

- The hips. These inside muscles include your inner thighs and pelvic floor.

Our strength-training component is another reason the Orangetheory workout helps members lose weight. Many of them do! But unlike many diets, where you lose muscle along with fat, **strength training builds muscle to help keep that metabolically charged body.** (My personal reason for continuing to work with weights in my late 50s is because I want to age well in my body. That's not going to happen with the hundreds of supplements that claim they will keep me young and vibrant. But it *will* happen with the weights I pick up and use during the weight-training rounds.)

Rowing: The Nonimpact Power Component of Orangetheory

As you saw in the previous chapter, I decided to include rowing as part of the Ultimate Workout to help create total-body power. As you age, your body's ability to generate power drops even more quickly than you lose strength.

"Rowing as a stand-alone exercise is unbeatable," says world champion rower and international fitness presenter Josh Crosby, who also serves on our Fitness Advisory Board. "It works nine major muscle groups, develops cardiovascular strength, increases flexibility, burns 500–1,000 calories an hour, and does so with minimal impact on the joints . . . . On top of that, using the WaterRower [a water resistance rowing machine] lends a feeling of authenticity and fun to the equation."

Besides developing power, rowing allows members to move and challenge their bodies in a unique way, says Crosby. "Many of the movement patterns we need to be better at in everyday life (especially as we age)—leg

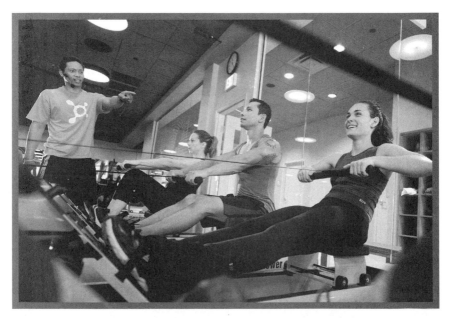

Rowing is a full-body exercise that develops power.

press, hip hinge, and scapular retraction [keeping your shoulders pulled back and down]—are combined by rowing into one integrated movement. This helps with posture, flexibility, and overall conditioning."

Another unique benefit to rowing is how you control the intensity. "With rowing, intensity is created by you, not a turn of a knob or gear change," says Crosby. "The harder you push and pull, the higher the intensity. However, because the workload is spread over all major muscle groups, the *perceived* rate of exertion for the participant is less. Simply put, folks burn as many calories rowing as they do running at the same intensity, but they don't feel as if they are working as hard to do so. In an Orangetheory workout, there is always an element of surprise. Rowing lends itself nicely to that. Rowing 300 meters is very different from rowing 1,000 meters, and you never know how the treadmill or weights will feel to you after jumping off the rower."

Published research confirms that rowing increases functional anaerobic power and all-over strength, which is why it's part of the Orangetheory workout.

Psychology: The Science behind the Brain and How It Works

When designing the Ultimate Workout, the number one priority for me, after it being physiologically sound, was the psychology of the concept. I knew that **making people of all levels of fitness feel successful** was a must. That became the basis of creating how the workout would be explained and coached.

What happens during an Orangetheory workout may not seem unusual to you, but the program has been designed to make you—and the person working out next to you—feel successful. That includes:

Giving a range of goals. When I started the Ultimate Workout, I would give members ranges instead of specific goals. So I'd say something like, "OK, now you're going to increase to Push by speeding up to about one or two miles over your Base," instead of, "OK, now you're going to increase

47

to one or two miles over your Base." This gave members some wiggle room and never set them up for feeling less than.

What never appealed to me about boot camp–type programs was that the design seemed to make participants feel like they were *not* doing enough. I wanted the opposite—I wanted people to feel like I appreciated the uncomfortable place they were putting themselves in.

Making people feel competent. My goal is that anyone who walks into an Orangetheory workout should feel empowered and successful regardless of fitness level. That's where the concept of Walkers/Joggers/Runners initially came from.

I knew that a group training format can go two ways. You can create an atmosphere with positive or negative reinforcement. I have taught and participated in thousands of group exercise classes in the past four decades, and I have seen plenty of classes where participants who didn't look, act, or do what the top 10 percent of participants in the class were doing were made to feel less than.

I knew that wasn't the atmosphere I wanted to create, because I wanted a program for all levels. I got rid of the word "modifications" in favor of "options." I never wanted Betty, who can't do a full-body push-up, to feel discouraged. So Betty has the option of dropping to her knees for a push-up. But I also created challenges for Joe, who's a super-fit 30-something. If he wants to kick it up a notch, he can do his push-ups with a clap in between. As both Betty and Joe become fitter, they increase what's called their self-efficacy, or belief in their abilities to accomplish tasks, and they can continue to choose the challenge that's appropriate for them.

Taking the focus off of the self. One of the things I never liked about group exercise was the natural drive to compare yourself to others around you. I knew women in particular were often discouraged or depressed when they were taught by a trainer with an extremely lean, toned body that they might not ever realistically be able to achieve.

So I created a large-group workout design where women wouldn't be staring at themselves in the mirror and worrying that their thighs were too fat or their arms were too jiggly. I wanted to get them out of the skinny mind-set and into the fitness and performance mind-set. So instead of worrying about how big their thighs might be, they'd feel great about how those thighs just powered them through an All Out at their fastest speed ever on the treadmill.

Using music for motivation. I've used music for 40 years as an instructor, teaching everything from dance aerobics to step. I know that research shows that music is a huge motivator and also reduces perceived exertion, or your own impression of how hard you're working out. It can also improve performance! Knowing this, I chose music with high BPM, or beats per minute, to help create high energy in the room, typically around 125–145 BPM. Music can also be a positive distraction during a Push or an All Out. Now at Orangetheory we vary the music to help appeal to people of all ages.

Behavioral Science: The Science behind *How* the Class Is Taught

After working on the physiological and psychological aspects of the program, the last part I needed to address was the behavioral aspect. What would keep my members coming back? One of the biggest problems in the fitness industry is member retention. About 40 percent of health club or gym members will drop their membership at the end of a typical year. I didn't want that to happen at my new studio!

So what was the answer? First off, I knew that I didn't want to ask members to devote their lives to improving their bodies. So I decided on a simple formula that members could do two or three times a week to get into shape, regardless of their initial fitness level. If a member's primary goal was weight loss, he or she could come three or four times a week. This formula made it very easy for members to know how much they needed to work out. It was all figured out for them.

I knew that the primary physical intentions of members joining a group fitness class were to get in shape, lose weight, achieve more muscle tone, and see changes in their bodies, so I took those intentions and created a formula that would meet them.

Using Orangetheory language. As part of the behavioral aspect of the class, I created what's now called Orange language. The goal of Orange language is to build members up, not tear them down. (Remember that's what I learned from my dad.) The routines are designed to help members continually move up and to see their improvements, whether achieving more Splat Points or noticing that their Base pace is now 0.6 mph faster than it was a month ago.

Making members feel special. One of the reasons people quit gyms is because they don't feel welcomed or never feel like they belong. We take the opposite approach at Orangetheory. We want every one of the 24 (or fewer) members at a class to feel special. That's one reason we ask Orangetheory trainers to give 10–20 personal touches per class. That might be using a member's name or acknowledging a job well done. That's part of motivating our members to **get comfortable being uncomfortable,** and it makes them feel part of the Orangetheory community—and that makes them want to come back.

One of the reasons I love the studio concept (as opposed to a larger gym) is that it is easy to personalize relationships and create a strong culture. Orangetheory members love being part of their culture. They wear T-shirts with our logos on them. They post about their workouts on social media. Some of them even have gotten our logo tattooed on their bodies! *That* is building culture, what we often refer to as the Orange Nation.

Consistent messaging. It was very important to me—and my partners—that Orangetheory maintain consistent messaging across all of its studios. So whether you go to a studio in Fort Lauderdale or Denver, Colorado, or Orange County, California, you know that you'll get a unique, metabolically charged workout, taught by trainers who use the same kind of language. That consistency (even while the workouts themselves are always evolving and changing) makes people feel comfortable and safe, especially when so many things about our lives can feel out of our control.

Constant change. Ever plodded away on a treadmill for 30 or 45 minutes? You were probably bored out of your mind. Well, at Orangetheory, you're constantly mixing it up. If you're on the treadmill, you may be changing pace from Base to Push to All Out, for example. Or you may be doing a power challenge on the water rower. Or doing four sets of challenging weight exercises before you head back to jump on the treadmill. It's one hour where you'll never look at the clock because of boredom, and that makes you want to come back!

Nothing Is Constant but Change

As I just said, boredom is a huge issue for most exercisers. You get bored, you lose interest, and you stop working out. We never want that to happen with our Orangetheory members, so we're constantly using the latest research to create new challenges for our members to keep them engaged and happy—and fitter as well!

Currently, we design 30 hour-long Orangetheory workouts every month, following our program and design parameters. When we roll them out, we're constantly collecting feedback from our franchisees, trainers, and members themselves to continually improve the quality and variety of the workouts and ensuring that you are unlikely to ever do the same workout twice—and that you'll never be bored!

Now that you know how the physiology, psychology, and behavioral science behind Orangetheory create results for members of all ages, you may be wondering . . . so what's it like, exactly? If you've never been to an Orangetheory class, you'll find out in chapter 4.

Orangetheory in Action: What to Expect at Your First Class

OK. So you're reading this book. Or maybe there's an Orangetheory in your neighborhood or you've driven by one on the way to work. Or maybe a friend or relative or neighbor is going to Orangetheory and raving about it. You're thinking, Maybe I could give that a try! But you're nervous . . . or worry you won't be able to handle it. My purpose in writing this chapter is to help you overcome any hurdles you have about walking through the door of your nearest Orangetheory.

Ready to Walk through the Door?

Ready? Here's what to expect:

Chances are you'll call the studio first to book a workout. The person you talk to should tell you to bring a bottle of water and a towel. He or she will also ask you to come 20–30 minutes before class to fill out and go over your intake form. Or you may just decide to stop by a studio to find out more about the workout.

Either way, when you walk into an Orangetheory studio, it feels like the TV comedy *Cheers*. You know, the show about a bar of the same name, where when you walk in, "everybody knows your name"?

Not only are staff members trained to know all existing members' names but also we actually have a Green Star signal on the computer so that the staff will know that you're new to Orangetheory and we can start creating a personalized experience for you.

The feeling of community and camaraderie is one of the first things to hit you when members gather in the hall before a class. Members are excited, not only for the workout but also to see each other and prepare together mentally for a great training hour.

But first we have to get you started. After you arrive, you'll fill out your intake form. An Orangetheory staff member will ask about your fitness goals, whether you are taking any medications, and whether you have

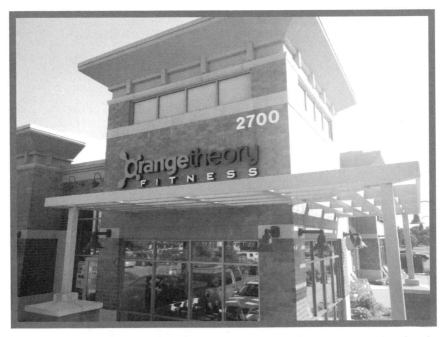

Every Orangetheory Fitness Studio has a distinct exterior look.

any orthopedic issues or injuries that may affect your ability to work out. Please be honest with the staff! This is to ensure your safety; our front desk staff will let the trainer know whether you have any current limitations. (The trainer for the class will also ask whether anyone has injuries or issues he or she should be aware of.)

The next step is to introduce you to our OTbeat heart rate–monitoring system. This starts the educational journey you'll be on for your first training hour. The front desk staffer will help you put on your heart rate–monitoring strap (you can borrow one for your first session) and the OTbeat monitor that snaps onto the front of the strap.

You'll be shown the OTbeat screens above the treadmills that will calculate (by what are called Splat Points) how many minutes you spend in the Orange and Red Zones. Your goal is 12–20 minutes by the end of the hour. If you haven't been doing cardio workouts on a regular basis, we'll suggest that you stay in the Green Zone for the first couple of weeks of training. When *you* feel you are ready to start delving into the Orange/Red Zones, then you go for it!

This is why Orangetheory is so unique. We address the not-training-hard-enough and training-too-hard issues most exercisers face. Remember the number one reason **why workouts do not work for most people is the intensity** (or lack of it!) and not knowing how hard is hard enough.

My Orangetheory:
It Makes a Great First Impression

I had heard nothing but positive things about Orangetheory, but I still attended my first class expecting more of the same—a packed class of ladies in rows in front of a giant mirror, desperately trying to either hide in the back or shame the rest of the class with their overly exuberant expertise. I expected to leave feeling I had spent half the class failing to follow a series of complex combinations and sweating over my embarrassment, not my workout.

> I could not have been more wrong! Despite being unfamiliar with the pacing or structure of the class, I found it easy to follow along. The class was packed with young and old, men and women, and all fitness levels. I was comfortable with all of the exercises and never felt like the "new kid" in class. I left feeling proud, excited, exhausted, and eager to attend my next class. Orangetheory makes a great first impression!
>
> —Jessica Klausner, 35 years old

Inside the Studio

Once you're set, you'll step inside the studio, which includes three areas—the cardio area, the rowing area, and the strength-training area. The cardio area includes 12 treadmills, one or two striders (or ellipticals), and one or two stationary bikes. The rowing area includes 12 water rowers. The strength-training area includes 12 TRX systems (these are the canvas straps that let you train with your body weight), and 12 weight-training stations. The OTbeat screens are located in the cardio area, and there is a visual aid screen in the strength-training area, which will show demonstrations of all of the exercises you'll perform and tell you how many reps (repetitions) to aim for.

All of the workouts are designed by the professional fitness team at the corporate office, using our ESP format. They are tested for results, and 30 new routines are sent to each studio every month. That means that every Orangetheory studio does the same workouts each day.

For your first workout, you'll start on the rower so you can start to acclimate to the stimulating environment. Your trainer will have you warm up and then coach you through your workout, suggesting three different paces: Base, Push, and All Out.

Your trainer will tell you that your Base is a moderate effort you can maintain for 20–30 minutes (this feels challenging but doable), Push is a more intense effort that you maintain for a shorter period of time (this feels challenging and is never more than three minutes), and All Out is where

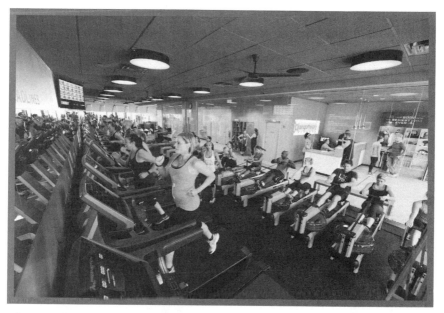

The cardio and rowing areas of an Orangetheory Fitness Studio.

you up your intensity to nearly as high as you can handle (this feels very, very uncomfortable but is only for as long as one minute, max). When you look at the OTbeat screen, the Green Zone is your Base, the Orange Zone is your Push, and the Orange/Red Zone is your All Out.

My Orangetheory: I'll Give It a Shot

I learned about Orangetheory from ads that had an orange tint. I also heard a lot of people talking about this workout where you used a heart rate monitor to see your progress and that it was a good, intense hour-long workout.

I'd tried a lot of fad workouts, and nothing seemed to be working, so I thought I would give it a try. I didn't have huge expectations—my goal was to be healthy. That was really my bottom line: I was not healthy. My triglycerides were high, and my cholesterol was high. I'd put on a lot of weight and had ignored that for several years. I'd tried several different workouts and even hired a personal trainer, but I wasn't making the connection I needed. I saw the ads for Orangetheory and thought, "I'll give this a shot."

I came in and liked the intimacy of the class; it felt like you were working with a personal trainer. What made the difference for me was that you have a trainer working with you but you're also able to see your own body do the work, wearing the OTbeat heart monitor, so you're actually watching your body respond to the workout.

Since my first workout, I've lost more than 60 pounds, a little more than a pound a week. . . . My doctor told me a year ago that I was going to need cholesterol medication. Now my cholesterol and triglycerides are completely in the normal range. I'm healthier, I feel better, and I have the energy you have when you *know* you're healthy.

— Chris Stotz, 38 years old

Depending on your current fitness level, your trainer may suggest that you stay at Base pace throughout the first workout, or he or she may have other suggestions for you. Your workout will include cardiovascular interval training, strength training for your outside muscles, strengthening moves for your inside muscles, and power training. The workout is for all levels—whether you're a Walker, Jogger, or Runner. You'll also have options in the weight room if you're concerned about your ability to perform an exercise.

After the workout, your trainer will lead the entire group through a brief stretching session; then, he or she will walk you over to the OTbeat screen to review your results. You will not be singled out or embarrassed; this is simply a tool for you to use to know what you need to do next time you train. (By the way, my neighbor, Crystal, doesn't even use her real name at Orangetheory! She makes up her own screen name, and you can do the same. Whatever makes the class a great experience for you!)

Just an hour later, you'll walk out the door feeling energized and proud of yourself. And I bet you'll already be thinking about coming back!

My Orangetheory: Hooked from the Start

I had been living in Orange County for about six months and was having a hard time fitting in or even finding a group of like-minded individuals. I had tried several fitness studios and large gym facilities, but nothing had satisfied what I needed. I saw an article on Orangetheory Newport Beach in a regional publication, and I immediately called the studio and booked my first class.

It had probably been about six months since I had seriously worked out. That was my pattern—work out for six months, and then take a break for six months. Nothing out there held my attention for a longer period.

My first class was a whirlwind! I was set up with a heart rate monitor, and I was a bit hesitant that my stats would be on a 60-inch screen to be publicly scrutinized. But I jumped on a treadmill and hit start. The music was invigorating, and the coach had a voice and energy that propelled me through the physically challenging class. I remember at one point looking around and being overwhelmed with the hard work and energy from everyone. I hadn't felt that way in months and was hooked.

Once the class was over, the coach reviewed my workout summary, and I was super proud because I had been in the red for the majority of the class. When he explained what my actual results should be, I regarded it as a challenge. . . . I talked about the class for days. With one simple phone call, I was a member, and that was over a year and a half ago.

Orangetheory has given me a lot of firsts. It's the first workout I haven't taken a break from after six months; it's the first workout where I haven't been afraid of lifting heavy weights; it's the first workout that I am using to train to hike the John Muir Trail with a 35-pound backpack; and, most importantly, it is the first place I have felt like I belong.

—Edie Trott, 32 years old

Frequently Asked Questions about Orangetheory

Q: I'm 65 years old. Is this class for me?

A: I just taught a class today that had a 70-year-old on the treadmill next to a Miami Dolphins football player. Due to Orangetheory's three categories (Walkers, Joggers, and Runners) and three intensities (Base, Push, and All Out), nearly anyone who is mobile can do Orangetheory. The All Out for my 70-year-old was power walking at 3.5 mph and a 3 percent incline, while my football player was running at 10 mph at a 10 percent incline. So, yes, if you're healthy and willing, why not give it a try?

Q: I'm pregnant. Can I still do the workout?

A: Obviously, you should check with your doctor first, but you should be good to go with some options. (I would not suggest Orangetheory to someone a few months into her pregnancy who hasn't been doing any kind of fitness training. Wait until after you have your baby and we can help get you back into shape!)

If you've already been doing Orangetheory and become pregnant, again, check with your doctor first. With your physician's OK, we believe our heart rate monitoring is a perfect way to keep an eye on your intensity as you progress through your pregnancy. I have witnessed my Joggers and Runners switch to power walking by the end of their pregnancies, but they've stayed very fit throughout! The TRX straps are a perfect option when you can't do floor exercises anymore, and your body will snap back after the baby.

Q: **I have bad knees and cannot jog. Can I do Orangetheory?**

A: I am with you on this one. I have arthritis in my knees due to those many years of aerobics, step classes, and running. The best part of this training format is you will never do more than an eight-minute block before walking it off. I'm 58 and have found the workout is very doable; on days when my knees ache, I used the strider or bike instead. The last thing I want to do is to stop moving my knees—they will stiffen up, and then I will really start losing my mobility! Remember **to do what you can do and don't worry about what you can't.**

Q: **My wife goes to an Orangetheory studio, and she is trying to get me to go, but aren't all the members women?**

A: Group training has had a reputation as a woman's form of exercise for many years, so I think some men still (wrongly) believe that. Group training isn't only for women. As a matter of fact, about 30 percent of most of our studios' members are men!

We think that in the next few years this percentage may easily be 50/50. This type of training can take a muscle-bound gym guy and make him look more cut, or defined. Many of our male members who lift weights continue to do their heavy weight training at the gym but still take their multivitamin workout twice a week! I have heard more than a few times how that has resulted in them being in the best shape of their lives.

Q: **Do I have to sign a contract to join Orangetheory?**

A: No. We have a noncontract policy. We're not interested in taking advantage of you during a vulnerable moment when you really want to get in shape or get healthier and lock you into a long-term contract. We are more interested in **proving ourselves on a daily basis**. We understand you may want to get into a workout routine, so one of our desk associates will offer to help you with that and show you how to prebook workouts for a month. If you haven't attended an Orangetheory class for a while, the Head Coach at your studio will follow up with you and offer you a private consult if you need one.

Q: Where do you find your trainers?

A: We look for student-based fitness professionals to lead our classes as opposed to teacher-based trainers, who make the workout all about them. Our trainers all go through vigorous, consistent training to ensure that they can not only coach and teach a class but also motivate, inspire, and encourage.

Q: Why are the workouts an hour long?

A: As I said earlier, lack of time is the number one reason people don't exercise, so our workout takes just 60 minutes. Members love getting in and out within one hour, and this training model gives you that multi-vitamin workout that you need in that time frame!

Q: Why can't I bring my iPhone into class? I may miss an important call.

A: As I said earlier in this book, we are on overload all the time. Taking an hour to "tune out to tune in" is good for not only your body but also your mind and spirit. The cell-free zone gives you an opportunity to turn off all of the day's stress and tune into your body fully in class.

Q: What's the deal with the orange lighting?

A: It's orange for a couple of reasons. First, it's Orangetheory. Second, Orange represents energy. But more importantly, the orange lighting was included to get away from fluorescent lighting! I've been under that fluorescent lighting for 40 years, and it doesn't make anybody look good. So the lighting is bright enough so that you can check your form in the mirror if you want to while still providing a softer ambiance. Members have told us they love the look.

Have other questions? Visit our website, *www.orangetheoryfitness.com*. But I would tell anyone who's curious about Orangetheory to simply come to a studio and try it. I think you'll be hooked!

My Orangetheory: I Instantly Felt Like Family

I've got to admit I was super nervous when I arrived for my first Orangetheory workout. I was greeted by the most energetic and welcoming trainers, instantly being made to feel like I was part of a family. Yes, the workout was intense, and, yes, at times I wanted to give in and give up, but I kept pushing because of the encouragement from the trainers, even getting to work out with the gym owner right beside me.

It's been a long time since I cried after a workout, but sitting in the car after the workout, I was overcome with a sense of pride and motivation to push harder, make myself a priority, and continue the fight to put my health and fitness first.

—Paul Jamison, 32 years old
(after his first Orangetheory workout)

Section 2

Beyond the Studio:
Orangetheory Lessons for Life

5

Base: Building Your Foundation

In Orangetheory, Base is a challenging but doable pace you can maintain for 30 minutes or more. As you know if you're an Orangetheory member, you have to be able to maintain Base before you can challenge yourself with a Push or an All Out. Think of Base as the foundation for higher-intensity exercise.

Well, the same idea applies to your life as well. One of the reasons I decided to write this book was because I realized I'd been applying some of the Orangetheory lessons to my own life and helped members do the same.

That doesn't mean I always *knew* that that's what I was doing at the time! When I graduated from college in 1979 with a bachelor's degree in physical education, I could not wait to teach physical movement to students. But I didn't find a permanent teaching job when I got out of school. Instead I was hired by the Niagara Falls YMCA to be the "on-the-road" phys ed teacher to area Catholic schools that didn't have phys ed programs. The YMCA had received a grant to make this happen, and I was hired to fill a van with phys ed equipment and hit one school a day, five days a week.

The kids loved me. They'd scream with delight when I pulled the van into their schools' parking lots. But talk about having to have vision! None of the schools had gyms, so I was running kids up and down school stairs. They ran around the churches, did push-ups against church walls (was that sacrilegious?), and played kickball games in the parish parking lots. One day one of the kids almost took out a nun at Sacred Heart Church!

We were in the middle of a very passionate kickball game, and no one saw Sister Catherine heading across the parking lot. A little girl kicked the ball in the air, and it headed straight for the sister. I yelled, "Sister Catherine! Look out!" I swear she went right into the Orange Zone that day!

I loved this job, but it lasted for only a year. I continued working for the YMCA for about five years and eventually became its director. While I was there, I wrote a grant that enabled me to create the first senior fitness program in Niagara Falls. I had nearly a hundred 65- to 88-year-olds who I taught three times a week. I also started what I called a one-bounce volleyball league for seniors in the city that was very popular.

Bela was one of my favorite members. At 88 years old, he never missed a workout class or a volleyball game—always while wearing his bowling shoes. For years I tried to get him into sneakers, but he refused. Oh, well— you have to pick your battles! I was getting him to move three days a week, so I was good!

I loved working at the YMCA, but by the end of the '80s, I'd had enough of the cold New York winters and wanted new opportunities. My husband at the time and my son and I moved to Florida, and I was hired by Bonaventure Spa. It was there that I feel like I really began to build the foundation for my fitness career.

I've always been a believer in doing my best, in large part thanks to my dad. Take the time when I was eight years old and my dad decided to enter me in an ice-skating race. I still have no idea why he thought this was such a great idea—I was nowhere near a seasoned skater. Yes, I could manage skating around the perimeter of the ice rink a few times, but that was it.

Remember that I'm from an Italian family, and there's something that occurs to Italian mothers—they're convinced that the cold will do something terrible to their children. So that Saturday morning, my mother packed layers and layers on me, with a pink snowsuit being the last outside layer. I barely could walk. My father had to help me put my skates on.

Eleven other girls and I lined up for the race. I looked to my right and saw Beth Coffee, looking lean and mean, wearing nothing but a tight fitted outfit and a hat. I was trying to manage this six-foot-long scarf wrapped around my neck about 10 times, hoping it would not hit her in the head while she was standing next to me. My father was off to the side, giving me this huge "You got this" smile.

The whistle sounded, and everyone took off, leaving me far behind. My steps were tiny, and my arms thrust side to side, scraping my snowsuit. Well, it did not end well. Not only did I come in dead last but also I believe they were picking up the cones off the ice as I crossed the finish line. Beth won the race.

My father was ecstatic. "You were amazing! You got around the corner *so* great!" He bought me my favorite candy bar—a Reese's Peanut Butter Cup—and I can still see the smile that was glued to his face. He was thrilled because I'd done my best. There might be only one winner, but if you always do your best, *you* will win as well. And Beth Coffee? Who knows? Maybe she became an Olympic speed skater or something.

A Small Fish in a Big Pond

What did it mean to be my best in Fort Lauderdale? I'd gone from being a big fish in the small pond of Niagara Falls to being a very small fish in a very big sea! I'd grown up in a modest middle-class family, in a middle-class neighborhood that was nothing like the area where I'd be working in Fort Lauderdale. But even before I moved there, I'd already decided I wanted to work for one of the best fitness facilities. I'd asked my sister, who already lived in Florida, for the names of the leading clubs because that's where I wanted to teach.

I'd never seen anything like Bonaventure before. It's a destination spa where movie stars, celebrities, and wealthy people would come and stay for a week to work out, eat well, and de-stress. Pulling onto the property, you're greeted with huge waterfalls and dramatic statues. On my first day, the smell of the herbs and potions for all the varied spa treatments was a whole new world to me. At Bonaventure, every client is given a huge fluffy robe, slippers, and a fresh workout outfit every day. Attendants carry all of the clients' personal items to and from their lockers.

This was my first experience with five-star service and where I first learned the difference between mediocre and excellent. From the first day I was there, I decided this would be the type of environment I would work in from then on out.

I was the exercise physiologist at Bonaventure Spa and wrote personalized home exercise programs for people to do when they went home. I'll be honest. At first I didn't feel like I belonged there. I was a small fish; remember? I was swimming against the big current, but from the first day, I was determined to become bigger. I decided to learn as much as I could about my profession as well as the wide variety of members I would come across.

In this new environment, I constantly felt like I had to prove myself. For me, that meant getting as much education as I could. I took every certification I could. I read trade journals. I attended every fitness conference that existed! I always believed that when I stopped learning, I would stop growing and I would lose my passion for the fitness business. (Well, 40 years later, I still haven't lost my passion.) When my husband and I divorced when my son, Evan, was two, that just made my passion and my drive to succeed even stronger.

While I was at Bonaventure Spa, I was offered an even better job at Williams Island Spa in Miami. Williams Island is a high-end residential fitness spa in a luxurious community that includes its own tennis center, restaurants, and a nearby golf course.

I managed the fitness area, the spa, and the beauty salon and had 50 employees working for me. There were about 800 members. I already had experience with five-star service, but here I learned that members would pay a premium price for a premium product or service. The key was that everything from the workout itself, to the music, to the instruction, to the cleanliness of the studio had to be next level.

I also learned that how I treated people made a huge difference in how they responded to me. In college, I'd learned about world-famous psychologist B. F. Skinner. His work showed that when animals were rewarded for good behavior, they learned more rapidly and retained more than those who were punished for bad behavior. I taught group classes with this mind-set and realized that if I criticized (even in a humorous way) someone or made a member feel less than, I would never get the best from that person. Although boot camps were becoming very popular during this time, the "that's-not-enough" mentality and bullying approach did not resonate with me.

Instead, I found that the more energy I gave to my members in my classes or at my fitness facility, the more I got back! My members would refer my facility to their friends and would stay with us for years. This energy kept me going. The best way to describe how I felt was when you volunteer somewhere, like a food bank, and you see how you touch lives and that makes you want to keep giving. I felt fortunate that my profession let me use my physical, mental, and spiritual energy to help improve people's lives.

During this time, I also found some wonderful mentors who would help me to develop skills that would carry me through the Pushes and All Outs of my life. I was fortunate to work with people who allowed me to focus on possibilities and opportunities rather than what is wrong—just like my dad did. Two of them, Richard Lamondin and Tim Nardi, also worked in the spa/fitness and hotel/fitness industry, and both served as mentors to me. Working with Richard and Tim, I learned a lot about how to be a great leader.

Both of them knew how to excite the people working for them, how to set priorities, and how to educate their staff about why they're doing things a certain way. Both of them motivated me to do more and taught me how to be a better leader. Great leaders have relentless focus, first, and they're able to take action.

As I gained experience and confidence, I found I was drawn to people like Richard and Tim—people whom I considered visionaries. Later I'd realize that these were the people who naturally Pushed in their own lives. (I didn't know then that I'd find three more visionaries in my Orangetheory partners.)

I also found role models in the fitness industry who were responsible for creating new workouts. I respected Jacki Sorensen, who created dance aerobics; Gin Miller, who created step aerobics; and Johnny G, who created Spinning. They were true visionaries who had the ability to create new fitness categories. (Once again, little did I know I'd be doing the same thing a few years in the future.)

Those role models I worked with and those in the fitness industry were truly inspiring, yet I found that a lot of fitness professionals didn't have much business knowledge. Or, they might know a lot about one area of fitness but lack knowledge in others. I knew I had the knowledge, and working with mentors like Tim and Richard, I learned that a good manager makes you feel respected, supported, and valued.

I also became more confident in my personal style of working with people. Ask anyone—I'm direct. But I'm also respectful, and people appreciate my direct approach. Over time, I also learned to listen to others and to be open to input. Nearly everything I was doing at these positions—teaching classes, managing staff, obtaining certifications, and even handling day-to-day problems—I now know was building my Base for what would come next: the creation of the workout that would eventually become Orangetheory.

My Orangetheory:
Words Cannot Explain What It's Done

Orangetheory Fitness is the best thing that has happened to me since I migrated here to the United States in 1991. This establishment has majorly impacted my life in ways words cannot explain . . . . I started going to Orangetheory in the summer of 2014 when I weighed a whopping 390+ pounds. And now today, in less than a year, I am down over 130 pounds. Attending the OTF classes is without a doubt the most significant part of the lifestyle changes that I made to get me where I am today.

I will wholeheartedly recommend them to anyone who wishes to transform themselves physically and health-wise. They will work with anyone at whatever level of fitness you are, and you are guaranteed results, provided you attend their classes at least three times per week and most importantly give your best efforts during the workouts. That's all that I did and continue to do and look at me now. Truth be told, I am somewhat addicted to these classes, and it's not just me. I know many other members who feel the same way.

— Donovan Williams, 51 years old

Building Your Personal Base

But what does this mean for *you*? How can you apply Orangetheory's workout elements to your life to create your own Base? I believe three critical elements develop a strong Base:

- Adopting a positive mind-set.

- Knowing your strengths and weaknesses.

- Finding role models.

Let's look at each of these in turn:

Adopting a Positive Mind-Set

I can't emphasize enough the importance of a positive mind-set if you want to be successful. You have to embrace a positive outlook, even (especially!) when people are trying to tear you down or things aren't going your way. And if you're a parent, this means helping your kids learn to do the same thing.

When my son, Evan, was five, he played T-ball. At the first game, he took off toward third base instead of first. The coach, a fellow parent, got all out of control and started yelling (at a five-year-old!). He continued to yell at his players throughout the game.

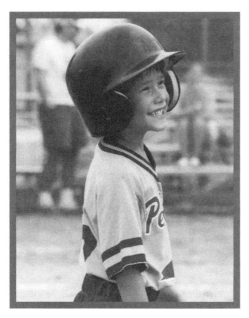

My son, Evan, at five years old.

Well, I'm sure you can imagine what I was thinking. But as the blood rose to my face, I (somehow) stayed in control. At the end of the game, I pulled him aside and tried to make him understand that yelling at a bunch of little kids wasn't the way to go. OK, I'll be honest; I got a little passionate about what I thought of his coaching skills. And I told him my son wouldn't be back. We found another team with a dynamo coach who understood that the way you coach is to build kids up, not tear them down.

Psychologists call your outlook your thinking style. My dad's thinking style was *your* personal best was your best. That's mine, too. But if I had continued to let Evan hear about his flaws and failures, I knew there was a good chance he'd create a bunch of "I Can't" channels in his head. (More about that in chapter 7.) Sorry, I'm not having it! I knew I had only one shot at being a parent, and I needed to do my best. So, bye-bye, Coach. (And I'm not bragging, but I think I actually did a great job. Evan is now a successful co-owner of two Orangetheory Fitness studios!)

We all have different thinking styles. What's yours? Are you more positive than negative or the opposite? Are you able to focus on what you have, instead of what you lack? If you want to explore your thinking style further, consider these questions:

How would you describe your thinking style, or your mind-set?

_____

_____

_____

If your thinking style is mostly positive, that's great. If it's not, think about how you can start to change it to a more positive one. What can you do? (For example, list things you're grateful for each morning; focus on what you already have in your life; take time to appreciate even minor things every day.)

_____

_____

_____

My Orangetheory: My Life Has Changed for the Better

After nearly 20 years with little to no exercise, I decided to join Orangetheory Fitness. I have significant health challenges as I am dealing with multiple sclerosis but wanted to improve my life at the most basic health level. I started my Orangetheory classes power walking and going three times a week. Within six weeks, I was off my high-blood-pressure medication and feeling improved.

After 30 classes, I moved up from walking to jogging, something I never thought I would do with all my balance issues. I am set to attend my ninetieth class tomorrow—six months in, and I have never in my life felt better. I still have challenges, but my physical fitness and cardiovascular health continue to improve and offset my illness. My coaches, the front desk staff, and all the members of Orangetheory form this incredible support network and empower me to continue to Base, Push, and All Out five times a week now! I have managed to run a mile in 8 minutes; row farther than I ever thought possible; lose 30 pounds and countless inches of size. I cannot wait to see what life is like after a year of Orangetheory, two years, and so on.

Within a doubt Orangetheory has changed my life for the better. I have never found a fitness plan I wanted to stick with, and I can honestly say I am addicted to Orangetheory! Buying clothes two sizes smaller than I used to wear is also a huge perk!

—Christopher Bradley, 37 years old

Know Your Strengths and Weaknesses

The second part of building your Base is knowing your strengths and weaknesses. My thinking style is one of my strengths. I also know that I'm great at inspiring and motivating people. That comes naturally to me. I'm able to get more from people than they ever thought they could do. I'm also willing to give all of myself in the moment, whether I'm teaching or working at my business.

But I have weaknesses, too. My lack of experience when I first moved to Florida was a weakness. I recognized that and tried to make up for it with more education, more certifications, and more knowledge. Although I may have gone overboard, I certainly turned what I had thought was a weakness into a strength—I learned a lot!

While I was working so darn hard (another certification, another book to read, another conference to attend), I did not believe in myself as much as I would have liked to. I consciously stayed safe. I wasn't much of a risk taker. I had this mega Base, but I was scared to go into Push. (Like a lot of new members at Orangetheory, I think I was scared to get uncomfortable.) While I did wind up getting pushed into Push (more about that in the next chapter), I wish I would have had the confidence to take more risks before that happened.

So what about you? What are your strengths?

_____

_____

_____

How do you use those strengths in your personal and professional lives?

_____

_____

_____

Are there ways that you could use them more effectively?

_____

_____

_____

Push

What about your weaknesses? What are they?

_____

_____

_____

How do those weaknesses get in the way of your goals?

_____

_____

_____

How can you address those weaknesses?

_____

_____

_____

My Orangetheory: Energy All Day Long

Since August 2014, I've lost over 50 pounds, and I've gotten incredibly stronger and faster . . . . Orangetheory has changed my life—the biggest way is the energy level I have now.

When I leave the studio, obviously I feel great, but the energy level stays with me throughout the day, so I get to go home and run around with my kids. And on the weekends, I'm out and about. I'm never still, and I never had that before Orangetheory . . . . I love the ability to see results, see the changes in my body, and see the way it's changed my life.

—Marissa Ames, 40 years old

Our Orangetheory: A Community of Support

Orangetheory has clearly been one of the most positive experiences of our lives. It's difficult to overstate the beneficial effects that this program has given to us: health, fitness, self-esteem, good friendships, and much more. The program demands a lot out of you, but it quickly delivers very positive and demonstrable results. . . . The structure of the program is one of its best features—the program is based on one-hour increments, and that makes it much easier to work into the course of busy workdays. When you put in that hour, you are guaranteed to have had an intense total-body workout. The program also generates significant positive mental results because of its focus on achievement of goals and commitment. It is difficult to quantify these mental benefits, but we have definitely experienced substantial positive effects such as increased levels of motivation and commitment (in and out of the gym) and more positive attitudes.

Orangetheory consistently has the best and most capable set of trainers. These folks set an extremely high standard of excellence and commitment in their classes at all times. They obviously care deeply about their role as trainers, and they push us hard to excel. We have been around gyms our whole adult lives, and we have never seen any set of trainers that even comes close to the Orangetheory team.

We did not go into the Orangetheory program expecting to make friends, but the positive social dynamics and the strong sense of support and community have become a vital part of the positive Orangetheory experience for us. We believe that this is one of the prime factors that sets Orangetheory apart from other gyms and fitness programs. There is a strong sense of mutual support among the members, and this continues to build as we attend sessions with the same people repeatedly and as new people join. There is also a very positive sense of friendly competition that drives us to excel, but this never rises to levels that would make people feel uncomfortable . . . . This is especially important to us as we are much older (ages 56 and 61) than many of the other members, but we are never excluded or looked down upon because of our ages.

One of the clearest indicators of the value and strength of the Orangetheory program is that we have stuck with it for five years now, and we have no plans to make any changes. Neither of us has ever stuck with another workout program or our own individual training for that long. The tremendous positive impact that Orangetheory has had on our lives is what drives this longevity. We both plan to stick with the program until we can't do it any longer!

—Terry and Bob White, 56 (Terry) and 61 (Bob) years old

Finding Role Models

As I said earlier in this chapter, I wasn't swimming against the current alone for long. Tim and Richard were both powerful role models for me. Another was my partner in life, Nick Granteed. Nick had built a very successful used car lot over the years. He had worked for himself all his life, and he was always asking me why I did not open up my own business. But that weak link of not being a risk taker surfaced, and I would have different excuses as to why I couldn't.

But Nick kept telling me, "There is no way you won't hit it out of the park! You're so dedicated!" In fact, he lent me the money to open the first Pilates studio in Fort Lauderdale in 2001, before I created the Ultimate Workout and opened my larger studio. In addition to people I knew personally, watching the careers of fitness pros such as Jacki Sorensen, Gin Miller, and Johnny G also gave me an idea of what path I might take eventually.

Role models can help you create a solid Base. You may already have role models in your own life, but if not, look around. Think about your goals and whom you already know who has qualities you admire. Your role models can be people you know personally or people you know of who are doing something you want to do or who are making choices you admire and would like to emulate.

Who are your role models?

_____

_____

_____

What about them makes them role models?

_____

_____

_____

What qualities do they have that you aspire to?

_____

_____

_____

How can you develop those qualities in yourself?

_____

_____

_____

Living in Base

For most of us, life in Base is challenging but doable—just like in Orangetheory. You may already be in Base without realizing it! It's normal to want to stay in Base—all of us want life to simply flow without many uncomfortable complications. Well, sorry, but that almost never happens!

Eventually, you're going to have an uncomfortable Push in your life. (Mine is coming up in the next chapter.) When your Base is strong, though, you're better able to handle the Pushes that occur. You don't fall apart and instead you actually become stronger than you were before. Embracing a positive mind-set, knowing your strengths and weaknesses, and identifying role models will help you build a Base that will help create the foundation you need to pursue your goals before you begin a Push.

6

Push: Getting Comfortable Being Uncomfortable

Last chapter, you learned about building your Base. Base is challenging but doable—like life sometimes. Well, what happens when life gets uncomfortable? That's a Push. That's when you have to learn how to get comfortable being uncomfortable. Learning to handle this discomfort is an essential skill not only during an Orangetheory workout but also in your life.

As I mentioned in chapter 5, it was never my intention to create an entirely new workout and fitness movement! But a number of things happened to Push me out of Base. The most significant was that I was let go from my job at Williams Island Spa in 1999.

When I looked at why I lost that job, I had to get real with myself. Yes, it was a dream job. I had more than 50 employees I loved working with. My position there opened a lot of doors for me in TV, including QVC, and magazines and newspapers. I'd become the go-to fitness expert in the Miami area. But I'd been there for six years and was a bit on autopilot. You know that feeling of "I've done all this before"? Ever feel that way in your job or in your life?

Well, that's about where I was. I wasn't in the gear that makes me the best version of me anymore. Around that time, I was talking with my friend Ed, who owned a Gold's Gym near my home in Fort Lauderdale. I had introduced Spinning to Williams Island Spa, but no gyms in Fort Lauderdale offered it yet. I subleased space from Ed and introduced my Spinning program there. It started creating a buzz. My employer became aware of it and felt it was a conflict of interest. That's why I was let go.

At the time, I wasn't exactly thankful for that, but part of what drives me is the limitless opportunities I have in my profession. *Today* I'm very grateful that I got Pushed out of my job; otherwise, I might still be there thinking, "It's a good job—don't risk it, Ellen." I wish I would have explored the distracted feeling I'd had for that last year or so, but I didn't. I was afraid. Fear is what makes most of us stay in the wrong relationship, stay at the wrong job, or stay around people with the wrong energy too long. The risk is what makes us fearful.

But if I had looked at my ultimate motivation, I might have realized that I wanted that next-level excitement and challenge. I've never been happy settling for the way things are. I'm always looking to move into a higher gear. I started Pushing myself immediately after the loss of this job by creating a Pilates business in a spare room in my house. About a year later, I opened Fort Lauderdale's first Pilates studio. The next Push—an even bigger Push—started when I signed the five-year lease on the building for the Ultimate Workout.

My Biggest Push Yet

This wasn't an easy time for me. But during this Push, I had an external sense of urgency. I had six months before the doors opened! This helped me be more accountable and procrastinate less. I also realized that I could create my own sense of urgency—an internal sense of urgency—to achieve my goals.

It took more than creating the workout to open Ellen's, though. When building out the studio that would house the Ultimate Workout, I surrounded myself with people who knew about the things I did not. I knew little about building a studio, but my friends Al and Jackie Fernandez, owners of ANF Construction, helped me find the location that would be Ellen's. They also took over every detail of creating the vision I had for the studio. For example, I didn't want florescent lighting—I wanted colored lights. I wanted high, open ceilings. Jackie and Al took my vision and developed the space that would later become the design for Orangetheory.

I also knew little about computers. I have to admit I didn't even use computers for several years at my Pilates studio. I checked in and billed members manually. But I found a computer guy, Dennis Cabrera, to help me with everything computer related. Dennis got me up to speed and never let me look back—and I'm thankful he's stayed with me for more than 10 years! Michael J. Schichilone, whose company is called Fitnessmith, was another resource I turned to. He guided me through all of my equipment purchasing and setup (and there was a lot of equipment I had to buy). He continued to work with me in the early years of Orangetheory.

After creating the workout and the place to do it, I focused on finding the right staff. I knew that the best leaders have dynamic personalities that resonate with both men and women of all fitness levels. Trainers become mini-celebrities at their studios, and I wanted individuals who were the best of the best. The class is the audience, so I started recruiting the best performers and created a pay scale that rewarded them for their talent.

My trainers were thrilled; they'd never made this much money at the gym by doing what they loved—training. And the members benefited as well. (A special thank-you to Casey Librizzi, Octavia Johnson, Bea Metz, Vinny Emanuele, Corey Summers, Bryan Spellberg, Nikia Hargis, John Driscoll, and Joyce Simmons for coaching the Ultimate Workout over the past eight years!)

If I wanted my members to perform, my employees to perform, and my business to perform, *I* had to be the best performer of them all. That meant I was in my studio 30 minutes before every class to prepare my music, review my workout template, and greet members.

In the early days I wrote hundreds of workout templates and kept each workout clipped to a clipboard. I wanted every member to love every workout and to rave about it to his or her friends! I quickly found that as long as my members felt like I was engaged and on this hour-long journey with them, they didn't care whether my timing was a little off or the flow was not spot on. They ended up loving the experience! Lesson learned—it's how you make people *feel* that matters.

Maintaining Focus during a Push

When you know how to handle a Push, the best part is that you are venturing into unfamiliar territory. It is having that leap of faith. It's like being on the treadmill at Orangetheory. You don't know what your Push will be that day, but you know you're going to go there. You start to understand the concept of **being comfortable when you are uncomfortable**.

I still felt that Push buzz when the doors of the new studio opened. I had committed my mind, focus, energy, and money to this project. Would I have enough money at the end of the month to pay the bills, to pay my staff? What about the competition?

I needed to continue to maintain that relentless focus. My dad would remind me to know what the competition is doing but to avoid putting energy into competing against them. Instead, I should use that knowledge to fuel my fire to go to the next level. I also didn't get distracted by rehashing decisions I'd made in the past. I've made some good decisions and some bad ones. I've tried to learn from the not-so-great decisions (like staying at Williams Island) and then move on.

To put excess energy into what is said and done is a waste of time and energy. I hate wasting energy, so I do not put energy in the past because I can't change it. I put a little energy into the future, which I have some control over. **The present is where I choose to exert my energy**. It's the only thing I have full control over.

But as I said in chapter 2, Ellen's was a success from literally the first day we opened on April 1, 2007. I believe that this was not only because of the workout itself and my fantastic staff but also because the studio itself was (and is) spotless. Cleanliness is a priority of mine. At least twice a day, my staff would clean the side railings of the treadmills, wipe fingerprints off of glass, and make sure the bathrooms and studio were spotless. Details are important when you want to be a high-end studio.

This was another lesson I learned from my dad. To say I was not the typical Italian daughter would be an understatement. When I was growing up, a "good" Italian daughter could cook up a mean lasagna dinner and keep the house spotless all day, even with a dozen children running around. My parents assigned all four of us kids chores from the time we were little, but I was never really interested in cooking or cleaning. I was usually trying to get out of my chores to go in the streets to play kick the can.

One day when I was about 10 years old, I was dragging a wet mop across the kitchen floor, in hopes of rushing out the door, when my father sat me down. He explained that what you put into something is what you get out of it. "Even though you may think mopping the floor is a meaningless job that doesn't matter, it does," he said.

He made an impression. When I finished, you could have eaten off of that floor! I felt proud of my work that day. I took that lesson—put everything you've got into everything you do—to Ellen's, and I do that today with my studio (I still own Ellen's) and with Orangetheory.

My Orangetheory:
Embracing the Uncomfortable

Orangetheory Fitness sparked a Push in my life that shifted everything for me—not just in the fitness room but also in life. Born and raised in the Bronx (New York City), I was comfortable operating my own fitness studio. After meeting Ellen and deciding to be a part of Orangetheory Fitness to share this life-changing workout with others, I had to change my life and move to Florida! I moved my family and left my home and successful business for the unknown.

It was very uncomfortable to relocate and to find a school for my son that provides the services he needs. The first six months were beyond uncomfortable, due to getting everything in order with my new position as the studio manager of Orangetheory Fitness in Cooper City, plus arranging my son's schooling and taking care of his home life!

One thing I learned from this workout is that Orangetheory Fitness teaches you to embrace the uncomfortable moments and Push through them. The workout is not supposed to be easy. Neither is life. The workout improves our lives by getting us outside of our comfort zones in order to make us healthier people. My life improved by taking a chance and welcoming the uncomfortable moments. This workout is not just an hour workout—it is a culture. A way of thinking. It can change your life when you embrace the meaning behind each step.

—Jai Faith, 36 years old, Orangetheory studio manager

My Orangetheory:
I Kept My Promise to My Daughter

Almost two years ago, I walked into a former fast-food location filled with Orangetheory gear, equipment, and team members who educated me about the Orangetheory workout. I was very intrigued by the concept, and so I joined, hoping it would be different from the other fitness centers I had belonged to in the past. That was the beginning of my life changing forever.

My marriage had ended, and I had a lingering promise that I had made to my beautiful, athletic daughter, Casey, who lost her battle to cancer at age 22. I promised to try to quit smoking and be happy and healthy. Well, I quit smoking, but I was neither happy nor healthy.

Orangetheory opened, and so my workouts began as a Walker on the treadmill, twice a week. Then I went three times a week and am currently a Runner attending four classes a week. I have never had the same workout, and I am always challenged during my workouts. I have lost 15 pounds, lost inches, and gained strength and muscle, and, yes, I now have "pipes"! I was able to run my first 5K ever in June 2015 in 31 minutes.

I have met so many amazing people who challenge me inside and outside of Orangetheory. What I did not expect was the mental and internal peace that I have achieved with my workouts at Orangetheory. I am forever grateful to the owners, Tim and Sherri, and the staff and amazing trainers for giving me back my Base, Push, and All Out in life and helping me keep my promise to my daughter.

—Deb Couture, 53 years old

Preparing to Push: Getting Comfortable Being Uncomfortable

You have to have a strong Base before you can Push. Once you have that Base, I've found that there are three elements to learning how to Push in your life:

- Maintaining relentless focus.

- Developing an internal sense of urgency.

- Getting support.

Maintaining Relentless Focus

When I think of the importance of relentless focus, I'm always reminded of my professor, Dr. John Piscopo, from SUNY (State University of New York) at Buffalo. Dr. Piscopo was my favorite professor. He was a small man who worked in the physical education/exercise physiology department with a lot of physical specimens. Despite his size, he stood out to me. My last semester getting my master's degree in exercise physiology, he said, "Ellen, your *focus* is what will separate you from others. So practice and get great at it." He worked with me on studying skills and helped me learn how to eliminate distractions and stay in the moment. His support and advice helped me get through my master's thesis!

Remember that I'm not a big risk taker. By launching my larger studio and creating the Ultimate Workout, I was venturing into the unknown. Would this workout and all the parts of it be a success? But in my gut, it felt very right. I was prepared. I committed my mind, body, and soul to this project. Sometimes you don't know how you're going to get there, but don't worry—if it feels right, *try*.

Part of maintaining relentless focus is to keep in mind what you can do and let go of what you can't. Don't worry about what others are doing, and don't compare yourself to others. **Keep working to be a better version of *you*.**

So how can you relentlessly focus? Start by identifying your goals, here:

_____

_____

_____

What steps do you need to take to meet those goals?

_____

_____

_____

Which step do you need to take first?

_____

_____

_____

How can you get rid of distractions when you're working toward your goals?

_____

_____

_____

My Orangetheory:
I Didn't Want to Be a Statistic

I'm a real experiential person, and I get bored with exercise quickly. What I liked at Orangetheory was the hands-on expertise of the trainers—and being in the class with people who were at different levels was inspiring.

I want to stay as mobile as I can—I worked for five years with people on dialysis, and a lot of people were there because they'd made poor health decisions and now they were attached to a machine for the rest of their lives. I didn't want that for myself. I didn't want to be a statistic, and I didn't want to take medication for the rest of my life. I may have one leg, but I'm able to get up and walk or climb a mountain or swim in the ocean.

If I'm not doing an exercise the right way, the trainers show me the proper way to do it—they don't let me slide, which I love, and they don't assume that I can't do something . . . . They recognize when I can do more, and when I'm in the Orange or Red Zone, my trainer will say, "Good job, Susan!" That means everything to me.

I never thought I could stick with exercise the way I have here, and because of that I'm starting to see some changes in my body I've never seen. Now I want to see how far I can go with this!

Before I started going to Orangetheory, I thought working out at the gym was boring, and I found a lot of excuses not to go. . . . I got into a real rut, which was work, stress, and ways of coping with that stress that aren't really all that helpful. I started to get concerned that my health was really failing, and I decided to make some really big changes in my life.

Orangetheory gave me all the tools that I needed to make those changes. I went full throttle in Orangetheory and began to push myself. When you push yourself so far, you begin to realize that you can really push yourself in any direction, whether you're at Orangetheory or outside Orangetheory. . . . I'm at a much better place because of it. I'm really focused on what matters in my life.

I'm focused on my dreams and my health, which is what I wanted to focus on. Orangetheory keeps me strong, focused, balanced, and energized.

—Susan Cooper, 48 years old

Developing an Internal Sense of Urgency

When I was creating the Ultimate Workout, I had an external sense of urgency that helped me focus. Well, you can create your *own* internal sense of urgency. I use this skill a lot. For example, I meet with my managers at Ellen's once a week, and we create specific goals for the next week and the next month. Everyone on the team knows what those goals are, who is responsible for them, and when they need to be accomplished by. They range from small goals such as "We need to change a lightbulb" to larger ones such as "We need to increase appointments by 10 a week." Before we meet the next week, everyone knows what he or she is expected to do, and if everything has been addressed, we can keep moving.

If you're the boss, or a manager, or even a parent, you can't expect high performance from the people around you unless you model and require that sense of urgency. Goals are great, but if I don't encourage my staff to take action, I'm not setting the example I want for my business. (We'll talk more about the importance of taking action in chapter 7.)

To create that internal sense of urgency, you set deadlines for yourself. Look at the goals you've identified above. Now, give yourself a time line to achieve each goal:

_____

_____

_____

My Orangetheory: I Learned to Push Myself

Orangetheory has changed my life. I'm not a professional athlete—I never was. I'm just a regular guy who grew up with weight issues that have stuck with me all my life. Always picked last for sports, never wanted to take my shirt off at the beach. I've tried every diet; I've tried every gym. Nothing seemed to work. I gain, I lose, and I gain it back again.

About a year ago I was more than ready to make a permanent change in my life. Thirty was around the corner, and I was tired of being embarrassed and not feeling comfortable with who I was. Around that time I got word that Orangetheory was moving into the neighborhood. I gave it a try and haven't looked back since.

The workouts were challenging; they gave me the perfect balance between cardio and weight training that I felt was lacking from other gym workouts. There was that feeling of community from the second I walked through the door. The staff was friendly, welcoming, and made me feel like I belonged.

Orangetheory isn't just a gym to me; it's become part of my lifestyle. I'm there every day pushing myself 100 percent just like the first day I joined. I'm now 30 and in the best shape of my life. I'm competing at a level with professional athletes. Without the constant support and motivation of the trainers, I would never have known I could push myself to achieve everything I have.

—Brent Gilinsky, 30 years old

Asking for Support

I will admit that I have a hard time admitting that I can't do it all. I used to feel bad about not being able to do it all! (Is that a woman thing?) But by accepting that and turning to others, like Jackie, Al, and Dennis, I found that I could focus on other things that I was great at. And if you want to make something great, not just good, surround yourself with people who will help make it great.

To relentlessly focus, you need people around you who truly care and support you. Nick was always there, propping me up. My sister, Cindy, and my brother-in-law, John Teeto, were a huge help to me as well. Evan spent a lot of time with them and their three sons, Johnny, Nicky, and Michael. They have also worked out at my studios and constantly recommend them to others. To this day, they're my biggest cheerleaders!

Take a few minutes and identify whom you can ask for support. List them here.

_____

_____

_____

What type of support do you need? Is it someone to watch your kids for a few hours so you can take a night class? A friend to brainstorm with and bounce ideas off of? A loan? Be specific about what kind of support would be most helpful.

_____

_____

_____

How will you ask for support? If your first choice is unable or unwilling to help, whom else can you turn to?

_____

_____

_____

Don't be afraid to ask for support and help from those around you. Most of us are willing to help someone else, especially someone we care about. Even simply asking for help can open the door for a stronger relationship between the two of you.

Pushing Past Push: What Comes Next?

Each of us will have times when we have to Push ourselves. Most of the time, when the Push ends, we settle back into Base. During that time, we're able to restore our energy and reboot. Then we can tackle another Push.

Sometimes, though, you may be challenged even further to Push harder than before—to go All Out. When you've learned to be comfortable when you're uncomfortable, you're ready for the biggest challenge of all.

7

All Out: Going from I Can't to I Can

After I opened Ellen's, my new, larger studio that housed the Ultimate Workout (along with other workout classes), in 2007, my business continued to flourish. Ellen's had three internal studios that included a Pilates studio with 18 machines that housed 55 classes a week; a Spinning studio with 32 bikes that housed 15 classes a week; and the Ultimate Workout, which had a capacity of 20 and housed 55 classes a week. We offered dozens of classes in a typical day, but the Ultimate Workout attracted the most attention and was very popular among members.

Many members lost weight or told me they felt like they were in the best shape of their lives. As word spread, the Ultimate Workout started to get noticed by people in the fitness industry as well. Local fitness consultants Bob and JoLyn Esquerre from Esquerre Group asked whether they could talk about the Ultimate Workout as part of their presentations at the International Health, Racquet & Sportsclub Association's annual conference in March 2008 and the World Spinning and Sports Conference in May 2008.

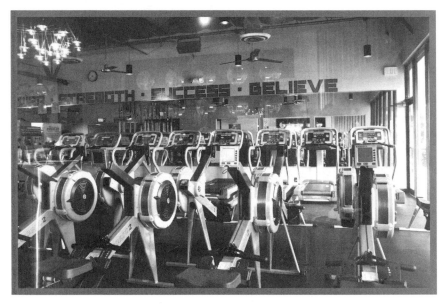

The rowers and treadmills at Ellen's.

Their sessions discussed how boutique, niche-based fitness businesses were becoming increasingly popular and successful. In fact, my studio was doing better business-wise than gyms that were three times my size! After the convention, quite a few gym owners came by to see what the noise was all about.

As I said last chapter, I had a vision of what I wanted the Ultimate Workout studio to look like. Painted above the mirrors on the walls are inspirational words such as "Believe," "Achieve," "Results," and "Success." When I sit in the front hallway of my studio, I can see directly into the Ultimate Workout studio and see the word above the mirror. In large letters, it reads "Believe."

One day in 2009, one of my members, April Kern, walked into the studio when I was sitting at my desk and told me I should talk to her husband, Jerome. "He does franchising, and your concept here would be great to franchise," said April.

I said something like, "I can't do that. I know nothing about franchising." That was the end of that, or so I thought.

At my studio, I often refer to our thoughts as channels. Sometimes the "I Can" channel is turned on, sometimes the "Maybe" channel is on, and sometimes the "I Can't" channel is on. I teach about 10 classes a week, even now, and before every class I tell my members, "OK, everyone check in up here to see what channel you're on," and I point at their heads. I'll continue, "I can't do anything with what's down here," and point at their bodies, "if you're not on the right channel."

We're not born with an I Can't channel. But somewhere along the way, someone—a friend, coach, teacher, parent, whoever—told you that you weren't good at something or that you wouldn't be able to do something . . . and you believed that person, and that I Can't channel got turned on.

You may think you can't change that channel. Years ago scientists thought that the brain was a rigid organ and it couldn't be rewired. But when they discovered something called neuroplasticity, they found that the brain is dynamic and adaptable. More importantly, it can be rewired! In other words, you can change your brain—no matter how old you are!

I've been in the fitness industry for more than 40 years. One of the reasons I've been successful is that I'm good at helping people see their potential, no matter how out of shape they may feel. That's why it was so important for me to create a workout for people of all levels—Walkers, Joggers, and Runners—and to have options instead of modifications. By offering a workout for all levels, I hoped that all of my members would feel *they* had potential to be able to successfully complete the workout. Believing in that potential and successfully completing each workout (or even completing a challenging Push or All Out) help change that I Can't channel to the I Can channel.

But remember that I'm not much of a risk taker. Fortunately, a week or two later, April came back into the studio. She hadn't given up. "You really should talk to my husband!" she said.

What was different *that* day was that I saw potential in the idea, and I took Jerome's number. (Later on, I'd realize that if I would have looked closely, I could have seen the word "Believe" on the wall behind April's head!)

I invited Jerome and his partner, Dave Long, to take one of my Ultimate Workout classes at Ellen's in the summer of 2009. Jerome and Dave owned a franchise development company, Ascente Corporation, and were looking for different concepts to franchise. They were both impressed with the workout and the science behind it, and we met several times to discuss the possibility of turning the Ultimate Workout into a franchise.

Dave had a fitness background and had the tools necessary to get the concept off the ground. As I got to know Dave, I found out he was the kind of person who liked to think things over before he spoke. I'm more of a think-as-I-speak type, and I liked the yin-yang relationship we were developing.

Jerome had already owned and run several successful businesses and was an area developer for Massage Envy. He had experience selling franchises, developing territories, and working with franchisees on a regular basis. I could tell from the beginning of our partnership that he didn't want to just create another franchise. He wanted each franchisee to be as successful as his other companies had been. One of the first things Jerome said was, "Ellen, I know that you're a highly passionate fitness person and that this is a cutting-edge idea. But I'm interested in franchising this concept only if it can be a grand slam for the franchisees."

Both Jerome and Dave were genuinely concerned about the success of the potential franchisees. I loved that. The other thing I noticed immediately about Jerome and Dave was that they were visionaries (something I aspired to) and risk takers (something I have struggled with in the past).

Jerome and Dave suggested that we add technology to the workout to provide immediate feedback to members. The three of us agreed that having real-time heart rate monitoring during the workout—and afterward—was key.

There was still a lot of fine-tuning to do, however. Before the pilot studio opened, we were building our brand, working on the price point for members, hiring staff, and developing training manuals and systems. We opened our pilot studio with room for 24 members in March 2010.

To prove how effective the workout was at helping people lose weight, Jerome proposed that we offer a weight loss challenge at the pilot studio. We agreed on a six-week challenge, and the winner of the first one lost an amazing 46 pounds. The tradition continues in every new Orangetheory Fitness studio. The resulting body transformations have been huge—members lose an average of 10 to 40 pounds during that time.

Dave, Jerome, and I welcomed one more partner, Dave Hardy, to Orangetheory a few years later. I first met Dave in 2009. Like Dave Long, he had experience in the fitness industry and had invested in different companies through his company, Franvest Capital Partners. Dave joined Orangetheory as a partner in 2012. Since then, he's been instrumental in helping Orangetheory grow from our first studio in 2010 to the more than 600 that have been sold as of the date of writing this (July 2015.)

Think. Speak. Be.

During the time we were fine-tuning Orangetheory and opening our pilot studio, I reached a whole new level of intensity. I'd Pushed before, but franchising the concept of my Ultimate Workout had my heart and blood circulating at an All Out pace! I was still teaching classes, managing Ellen's, and working with my partners on the franchise concept. I was playing on a bigger playing field than I ever had before, and I was in an entirely new gear—an All Out gear—than I had been before. I had very uncomfortable moments, but I also reached a higher level—just like in the workout.

Fortunately, the inspiring words of a yoga instructor of mine, Christine J. Lewis (president of Soul Foundation), resonated with me during these All Out moments: "Acknowledge that everything you encounter is actually strength and conditioning work to prepare you to create the life you want.

And anything you do consistently becomes a constant in your life," she told me. "If success and results are what you choose, then consistently focus on that in the way you *think*, the way you *speak*, and the way you allow yourself to *be*."

Think. Speak. Be. Focusing on how I do those three things kept my I Can channel turned on during these demanding times, and it helped me open my mind, body, and soul to living a life that had more potential than I had ever imagined. Today, I believe that **continuous improvement is the goal when it comes to All Out success**, whether you're talking about being a parent, partner, or business owner.

Orangetheory helps members reach for that continuous improvement. One of the reasons so many people have changed their bodies—and their lives—with Orangetheory is that it's an optimistic workout. Thanks to the structure and design of the workout and the motivational, inspiring coaching, members (even new ones!) focus on the possibility of success. You're focusing on what you're doing right, or well, instead of what you're doing wrong.

The physical challenges that the workout contains give members an opportunity to feel that continuous improvement. When you're able to hold a Push for three minutes, you feel a sense of accomplishment. When you go All Out at your highest speed ever and then walk it off, you're taking action. You're progressing. You're improving. You're becoming the best physical version of you. I call that striving for excellence.

You know from the last chapter that I'm committed to excellence in all areas of my life. I set an expectation of excellence for myself and how I approach everything Orangetheory—from my corporate position, to how I train coaches, to how I coach my own clients. By doing this, I lead by example and require the same level of excellence from those who work with me—from regional trainers, to head trainers, to coaches, to members. I believe people aspire to be their best when they are trained by people who *expect* their best.

Many people live mediocre lives. But that's not what I want for myself or for my members! By going All Out, at least occasionally, you, too, are striving for excellence not only during your hour at Orangetheory but also in the rest of your life.

My Orangetheory: Living Life at Base, Push, and All Out

I was diagnosed with stage 1 esophageal cancer in December 2013. I was shocked—how could this happen to me? I was a very healthy, very active 43-year-old woman.

Confronted with my diagnosis, I immediately went into a Push pace. I tried hard to keep everything in perspective and to learn and absorb as much information as possible about my situation. I also needed to keep it together for the sake of my 16-year-old son and 10-year-old daughter. From this, my darkest point, I got lost in my workouts and a positive mind-set.

I became more inspired in my coaching. I kept reminding myself that I was absolutely fine . . . except for the need to get the cancer cut out of my body. Tests determined that the cancer had not spread, and that was good news that fueled my determination to become as strong as possible before my surgery. Each day I had to tap into that uncomfortable Push pace mind-set, which always got me through. I took Orangetheory classes four times a week and went into my surgery feeling stronger than ever physically and mentally.

On February 3, 2014, I had a full esophagectomy, where doctors removed my esophagus and used my stomach to rebuild a new one. I was in the intensive care unit for three days and in the hospital for four more. I woke up with a 10-inch incision in my stomach, a three-inch incision in my neck, two drainage tubes, and a feeding tube. This was my All Out, and I had no other choice but to finish.

Once I got home, I hit Base pace. Everything was doable but challenging. I started walking each day, and after two weeks home recovering, I reached my first goal of walking two miles. My big goal was to get back to teaching Orangetheory classes four weeks after being released from the hospital. That seemed so unattainable at times, but I just stayed steady at Base pace, and, sure enough, I did it! After just four weeks home from the hospital, I was back to coaching some of my classes. But this was really just the beginning of a longer road to full recovery.

I etched in my mind that I would wake up every morning at Base—doable but challenging. Every afternoon became a Push/All Out as I attempted to get back to everyday life. As I would eat throughout the day, I would experience severe intestinal cramping, and it was very uncomfortable/miserable. But it would always pass, and I'd be back at Base—doable but challenging. It took eight months for me to feel 90 percent better, but each day I progressed little by little, and I never looked back.

The encouragement, love, support, and concern shown to me by my Orangetheory family were overwhelming. It's now one year since my diagnosis and 10 months since surgery, and I feel incredible. I can't say this strongly enough—Orangetheory is not just a workout. Orangetheory is a mind-set that will carry me through life.

—Melanie Cassitta, 45 years old (Orangetheory head trainer)

Preparing to Go All Out: Going as Hard as You Can

Learning how to be comfortable being uncomfortable enables you to Push. Going beyond that effort—giving it everything you have—is your All Out. I believe there are three elements to learning how to go All Out in your life:

- Seeing potential.

- Taking action.

- Striving for excellence.

Seeing Potential

Many of the people at Orangetheory already know how to switch the I Can't channel in their heads to the I Can channel. I do it every day in my work with people's bodies. I get people to believe in their own potential, and that helps them be willing to take action. I see this happening at Orangetheory as well—my partners, our franchises, our head coaches and trainers, and even our members are leaning how to do that. Our collective belief in Orangetheory has brought the company to an All Out status.

But what does that mean for you? How do you recognize the potential in yourself?

_____

_____

_____

List one area of your life where you know you have potential.

_____

_____

List one thing in your life where you would like to see potential—or express the ability to change in a positive way.

_____

_____

_____

(If you like, you can list other things in your life where you'd like to see potential.)

My Orangetheory: I Was a Ticking Time Bomb

Before I joined Orangetheory Fitness, my doctor told me I was a ticking time bomb. I was a prime candidate for a stroke and/or a heart attack. Since joining Orangetheory, I have transformed my body and renewed my personal motivational outlook.

In less than one year, I've lost 60 pounds and no longer need medication for high blood pressure or to manage my blood sugar, and I feel better than I have since I was in my twenties. When asked, "What's the secret?" I simply tell people, "No secret. Hard work, dedication, and workouts at Orangetheory!"

I'm 52 years old and tell everyone it can be done. I am now going All Out in my life the way it was intended to be lived.

—Al Silva, 52 years old

Taking Action

The biggest reason that people aren't living the lives they want is they fail to act. We talk about making decisions, we think about them, we ponder, we ruminate, we obsess . . . but we don't actually *do* anything!

To achieve your full potential, you must take action, and action starts and stops in the brain. In his book *Brainblocks: Overcoming the 7 Hidden Barriers to Success*, neuropsychologist Dr. Theo Tsaousides identifies the seven ways your brain can block your ability to express your full potential, thus preventing you from reaching your goals. The seven brainblocks are self-doubt, procrastination, impatience, multitasking, rigidity, perfectionism, and negativity:

- Self-doubt is a result of not knowing how to handle fear. Often, your automatic response to fear is to stop and freeze. You take no action, so you get no results.

- Procrastination is a result of low initiative. You're simply not motivated enough to do whatever it is you need to do.

- Impatience is a result of poor impulse control. You want something, and you want it *now*. So you take action without planning, without preparing, and without thinking through what you're doing.

- Multitasking is a result of insufficient focus. For the brain to learn a task—and execute it well—you must give 100 percent of your attention to the task. If you become distracted, your performance ability drops significantly.

- Rigidity results from lack of mental flexibility. You think only in terms of black and white, right or wrong, or "my way or the highway." You're unwilling to listen to advice or respond to feedback about your choices.

- Perfectionism is lack of prioritizing. Your brain loses track of the main point and focuses on unimportant details.

- Negativity results from a failure in reasoning. You make conclusions based on biases and beliefs instead of evidence. When you are biased, you look only for the facts that support your beliefs. If you believe that you'll never reach your full potential, you'll find reasons to support that belief.

Dr. Tsaousides's research gives us some very specific guidance on what holds us back. I wanted to create a workout that would help people overcome fear and that would challenge people not only physically but also emotionally. So the workout is designed to help you overcome fear and beat self-doubt along with other brainblocks. For example, you focus on performing one task at a time, so your brain doesn't try to multitask. But most important of all, you're taking action by showing up at Orangetheory. Every time you complete a workout (in fact, every time you complete a block, or a section of the workout), you're taking action. That helps overcome these different brainblocks and sets you up for success.

To take action in your own life, look at the answer you gave above—something in which you'd like to see potential in your own life.

_____

_____

_____

Now write down what you will do to take action on this area of potential this week.

_____

_____

_____

Striving for Excellence

When I hired the first trainers to coach the Ultimate Workout, I was looking for the best I could find. That meant trainers who were **striving for excellence**. If they're not striving to become the best _they_ can be, how can they set the example for others? I'm fortunate to work with some standout Orangetheory Fitness people who have helped all of us Push and accomplish some All Out moments, including Chan Gannaway, Orangetheory's education director; Barb Moylan, our regional and head training director; Corey Summers, our template design director; Clara Assael, template designer; and Jhoel Gaona, regional fitness trainer. They are the kind of people I want at Orangetheory and in my life!

When you go All Out at Orangetheory, you are Pushing yourself as hard as you can. That is striving for excellence! To go All Out in your life, list one thing that you have done at an excellent level during the past three months:

Now list another thing you'd like to do at an excellent level:

My Orangetheory: It's Made Me Love Myself

I remember walking into my first class on January 4, 2013. I didn't know then that this would change my life forever. I remember thinking, "This is impossible. Will this ever get easier?" After my fifth class, I remember telling my trainer and saying, "Thank you for changing my life." I remember him saying that it was my dedication in the classes that changed my life. His words inspired me so much.

Persevering through the next year almost every single day inspired me to Push myself past what I even thought possible. Since then I have run about seven marathons and four ultra-marathons, one being a 50-miler. Who would have thought that a New Year's resolution to take an Orangetheory class could change my life so much?

It's given me a love and passion for fitness that I never knew existed inside of me. And better yet, it's made me love myself! I'm a pediatric ICU nurse, and as most know, my job can be extremely sad and stressful—I have so many emotions to deal with in my career.

Orangetheory has almost been my "calm"—my sanctuary to go where I can get my butt kicked and clear my mind at the same time . . . . I can honestly say I'm addicted to Orangetheory Fitness!

—Jade Gaona, 31 years old

What Does an All Out Life Mean?

My father always emphasized education, and that's one way I have always kept ahead of the curve in my profession. When you live an All Out life, you continue to educate yourself. Invest your time, money, and energy in advancing yourself, whatever that means for you. Continuing to find better ways of doing things is what you need to do to go All Out in your life.

If I hadn't continued to study exercise science and had the desire to keep pushing the envelope with my knowledge, I wouldn't have been interested in developing a new workout. I would have just kept doing what everyone else did! It's the same for our lives. Whether you want to be a better partner, parent, employee, or employer, never stop learning. Attend workshops and conferences. Connect with others. Read. To live an All Out life, you have to have the desire to improve your game—and to always want to keep getting better. Embrace that desire and feed it and you'll live your own All Out life.

My Orangetheory:
I'm Living Proof That It Works

I won my Orangetheory's Grand Opening Weight Loss Challenge—I lost 22 pounds in six weeks, and I feel amazing! Life is busy, and making good nutritional choices and finding time to work out are difficult. With Orangetheory, I feel like I have a secret weapon that I want everyone to know about. The workouts are research based and incredibly motivating. The group personal training environment is part friendly competition and completely "mindless" at the same time. I show up, and the expert coaches tell me what to do every step of the way. My role is to monitor my heart rate on the posted screens to make sure I'm working in the right zones. The hour is up, and before you know it, I've worked my butt off, and my endorphins are racing.

I love seeing all shapes and sizes in the class and that everyone is focused on their own workout yet supportive of one another. These workouts are a challenge for everyone, from competitive athletes to newbie exercisers with 100+ pounds to lose; in fact, it's the new people, who are so committed and hardworking, who inspire me most.

I've worked out and have been a member of many gyms over the years. Orangetheory is different—they care about all members showing up and benefiting from the workouts because they believe so strongly in the results they see. Your job is to show up a few times a week for an hour, follow the instructions of the phenomenal trainers, and work hard. It's that simple—it works, and I'm living proof!

—Stephanie Brundl, 45 years old

Stephanie Brundl is more than just an Orangetheory member—she loved the workout so much she bought a franchise with her friend and Orangetheory member Connie Byrne. Next chapter you'll hear from other members who have taken the step to become franchisees—and how the Orangetheory movement is taking off!

8

Orangetheory, the Movement: The Growth of the Franchise

When I came up with Ellen's Ultimate, I didn't intend to create the workout that would give life to one of the fastest-growing fitness franchises. Nor did I have any idea five years ago when we launched Orangetheory that it would take off the way it has. But as more members have discovered us, there's been a corresponding increase in the growth of Orangetheory franchises. In 2011, there were 12 studios open; in 2012, we awarded 72 more franchise licenses. By 2016, we will exceed 500 studios worldwide. At this rate we plan to have 1,000 studios by 2018! Wow!

While I didn't know a lot about franchising at first, I learned fast. And my partners, Dave Long and Jerome Kern, have more than a 10-year track record of extraordinary franchise development with notable brands such as Massage Envy and European Wax Center. Thanks to their work, and that of Dave Hardy, Orangetheory has become one of the fastest-growing franchises in the United States. The company has expanded from the United States into Canada, England, Australia, and Colombia, and we're talking about more international locations now.

"Franchising has exploded across sectors and increased in sophistication. Each franchise comes with a ready-made formula plus resources, training, and people to guide you along the way," says Dave Long, Orangetheory CEO. "'Business in a box' is what it's called: open the box and make money."

However, there are plenty of franchisors out there who care little about the success of their franchisees. "The worst franchisors sell a dream and provide little in the way of substance and support. Meanwhile, they are collecting 5 to 10 percent or more in gross revenues from royalties. We are the exact opposite because we view franchisees as our partners. We know their success is inextricably linked to our success. We are relentless about providing them all the right tools and giving them a robust brand platform as a diving board into success.

"The reason Orangetheory 'blew up' is because the workout works for everyone. We created a fantastic brand around that. We brought the right franchisees on the team who are as passionate as the leaders of the company," says Dave. "We refer to our franchisees as the 'lighter fluid,' or the Orange passion, that has fueled our movement. The franchisees' caring attitude and the extra initiative they take to hire the best staff, keep facilities spotless, and always put the customers' needs first make Orangetheory stand out from our competitors."

In addition to having a unique franchise concept, Orangetheory provides plenty of support to its franchisees. "We provide a 360-degree platform that includes our scientific fitness program and how to deliver it," says Dave. "The details that make it successful are built into the processes provided to the franchisee to execute. A tremendous amount of technology monitors the system, and an entirely different technology platform is provided to the end user. Our franchisees drive the business; they are passionate and can build a world-class team to execute the business model. The most important part is that they all believe in the Orangetheory product."

In fact, we estimate that close to 90 percent of our franchisees were studio members first! When I created the Ultimate Workout, I knew that the people I hired to coach the workout were critical to its success. They needed to be pursuing excellence in their own lives to inspire and lead members to do the same. What we've seen in the past five years is that the same applies to Orangetheory franchisees as well. I've met many franchisees personally. I love getting to know them during the corporate training week. Listening to their stories, I can already feel the Orange passion beginning to build.

What Does It Take to Be a Franchisee?

Typically, about one person in 50 who expresses interest in franchising goes on to become a franchisee. We're four times more selective at Orangetheory; only about one person in 200 qualifies as a franchisee. We don't solicit for franchisees; they come to us.

We look for people who:

- Believe in the Orangetheory workout and the brand.
- Will commit the time and resources to develop a successful studio.
- Will build and nurture a world-class studio leadership team, including their head trainers and studio managers.
- Will follow the Orangetheory franchise system, which is proven to work.
- Will work as a team and protect the brand.

A potential franchisee typically contacts us through the company's website; we pride ourselves on reaching out to people within 24 hours. Then the candidate takes the following steps:

1. The candidate fills out an application and receives the franchise disclosure document. The FDD explains the nuts and bolts of the franchise system including the costs, training provided, and each party's duties.

2. Candidates participate in a monthly webinar hosted by Dave Long, Jerome, and me. We usually have about 200 on this call.

3. Candidates can also attend another webinar hosted by franchisees with open studios to ask questions.

4. An Orangetheory area partner, or local support person, interviews the candidate to determine whether the candidate meets the financial criteria and has the Orange passion to move forward.

5. Once candidates qualify and are on board, they have a robust technology platform and e-learning along with support from corporate headquarters in their local market. Candidates attend a full week of training at corporate headquarters and monthly webinars on fitness, sales, operations, and marketing. We give franchisees every tool they need to run successful studios from the time they start build-out.

Every franchisee's story is unique. Rather than make generalizations, I reached out to several Orangetheory owners and asked them to share their stories. Marc Thomas was the franchisee who turned over every rock before he came on board. I was impressed by how he researched every aspect of our business.

My Orangetheory:
I Feel Like I'm Doing What I'm Meant To

A wise man once told me that the ultimate career goal should be to align one's job with one's passions in life. Most people work for a large portion of the waking hours of their life, so wouldn't the world be a better, happier place if everyone could make a living spending all those hours doing something that he or she truly loves? It seems like such a waste of our limited time on this earth just going through the motions in jobs that don't stir our souls or motivate us to strive for greatness. When people do what they love—what they are passionate about—they cannot help but achieve success and, more importantly, fulfillment.

I know this to be true, but getting there is easier said than done for most. Three years ago, I was at a crossroads in my career. I'm a workaholic by nature and had always found success in life in whatever I was doing, but after nearly 18 years as a serial entrepreneur in the high-tech industry, I had lost the passion for it that once had motivated me and fulfilled me. I was ready for change, but I wasn't sure where to turn next.

I have always had a passion for fitness in my personal life. I was a multisport athlete in my youth, and as an adult, I spent many years as a competitive amateur runner, cyclist, and triathlete—with multiple Ironman triathlons under my belt. I was admittedly naive about the fitness industry as a career path, and I frankly didn't think people really made much money in fitness, so every time I considered it as a career option, I shied away.

Yet I was desperately seeking personal fulfillment in my career again. I wanted to look forward to going to work in the morning. I wanted to build something special. I wanted to improve the world around me. I wanted to be in control of my own destiny. I wanted to establish a legacy. I wanted to make a difference.

So after living in South Florida for nearly 17 years, I decided to move back to my native Southern California and begin the next chapter of my life. I got married in April 2012, and my wife, Stacey, immediately thereafter became pregnant. Right around that time, my good friend Jim Cahlin (now an Orangetheory franchisee) called me from Fort Lauderdale and said, "Marc, Orangetheory Fitness is franchising their concept, and they are blowing up out here in Florida. All the members I know are totally addicted. Maybe we should consider opening up a studio in California. I can arrange a call with one of the founders of the company. What do you think?"

I was vaguely familiar with Orangetheory Fitness since the original studio was only a couple miles down the street from my former home. I had a number of friends who went there regularly and raved about it. However, my initial reaction was, "What do I know about the fitness industry? And how would I effectively compete here in Southern California—the world's fitness epicenter—with a new, unknown concept? Surely, all the people who've already been in this business for many years have a much better chance at success than I do. This sounds awfully risky." However, I was also very intrigued by the opportunity to follow one of my passions and to maybe, just maybe, be able to make a career in fitness. So I agreed to make the call.

A few days later, I spent about 45 minutes on the phone with Jerome Kern, the cofounder and president of Orangetheory. What he told me about Orangetheory was incredibly compelling, and by the time the call was over, I had a radically different perspective on this nascent company's potential for growth and the magnitude of the business opportunity for me as a prospective franchisee. I had a fresh understanding of the lifestyle that it could provide me and my new family. I also felt that being part of this company could be personally fulfilling on multiple levels. I went home that night and announced to Stacey, "I think I figured out what I'm going to do with the rest of my life!"

The company was still quite small at that point in the summer of 2012. There were about 20 open studios and fewer than 10 people working in the corporate office, all of whom I met on my first visit. I toured quite a few of the studios, met with owners and staff, and asked tons of questions. (Jerome still ribs me to this day about how many questions I asked.) But everywhere I turned, the feedback was nothing but positive.

My gut told me that this was the right move, but I was still nervous. After much deliberation, I finally took a huge leap of faith: I took my life's savings and committed it to my future with Orangetheory Fitness. I was confident enough in the opportunity that I not only purchased a couple franchise licenses but also bought the exclusive franchise area development rights for Orange County, California. I went All Out!

My team and I opened the first Orangetheory studio in California in Newport Beach in January 2013. It was an instant hit. Word spread like wildfire around the region that Orangetheory Newport Beach was the place to work out. Some members were driving over 25 miles each way several times per week to take classes at our studio. Our membership grew at record pace. We were profitable in our first full month of operations, and our monthly revenue numbers quickly outperformed the projections in our business plan.

On top of the studio's rapid growth, I originally thought it would take me three years to sell all the franchise licenses in my region, but instead I completely sold out the territory in fewer than six months. Today, I own two open studios, have a couple more in development, and oversee seven open studios in my Orange County region. We will at least double that number of open studios in my region by the end of 2016, and I expect to own half of them.

And if that wasn't all good enough, nine of my close friends who attended my wedding in 2012 have since left their successful careers in various fields to open Orangetheory studios. Like me, they all followed their passions for fitness and now couldn't be happier to be part of the Orangetheory family—and I couldn't be happier to share the Orangetheory experience with all of them.

Orangetheory Fitness has changed my life forever in more positive ways than I can count. I am so grateful to Ellen, Jerome, Dave, and Dave and the rest of the Orangetheory team for the vision, the opportunity, and the support. It's been a tremendous blessing for me and my family. I truly feel that I'm doing exactly what I'm meant to be doing—as if it were my destiny to be here at this time, in this place, with this company and these people. I feel as if all the skills and experiences that I acquired in my 18-year career prior to Orangetheory were preparing me for this opportunity so that when it crossed my path, I would be able to recognize it, seize it, and fully appreciate it.

> I'm passionate about Orangetheory Fitness and what it stands for. I'm surrounded by people whom I respect and enjoy and who share common interests and goals. I feel an obligation to contribute in the best way I can to its success. Orangetheory is where I belong. I am truly fulfilled.
>
> —Marc Thomas, Orangetheory franchisee
> with studios in California

The next franchisee, Mike Singer, was a fellow fitness professional who had to overcome his fear of partnering with a franchise. Now we're family:

My Orangetheory:
I'm Finally Playing in the Big Leagues

When I was a kid, I played baseball. At seven years old I was the best kid in the whole league. I thought I was the best, and I was told I was the best. I really was the best! By age 12, some of the other kids were catching up to me. By the time I played high school ball, the competition had gotten pretty stiff. I was no longer the best on the team, and maybe I was just considered average.

I never had to work hard to be good at baseball. I just relied on natural ability, but I had learned a hard and painful lesson. The kids who had worked hard their whole lives to be good flew right past me when we got to the levels that really mattered. They had a stronger work ethic than I did, and they never gave up. In retrospect, this lesson was a real game changer for me. It had a huge impact on what eventually became my real future—my career in health and fitness. I went to the University of Texas–Austin, got a degree in kinesiology and exercise physiology, and moved back to my hometown, Miami, Florida, ready to work hard, never give up, always strive to improve, and never blow another opportunity because someone else had a stronger work ethic than me!

At the age of 22, I found fitness. I spent one year working in a community fitness center, built up a personal training clientele, and followed my gut and my heart! I had no knowledge of how to open a business, nor did I have anyone guiding me. I just saw an opportunity and used lots of common sense. In 1994, at 24, I signed my first lease and opened my first business, a personal training studio called Only You. I was so happy just to be able to make a little bit of money after we paid all the bills.

Two years later, with 20+ trainers on staff, we moved to a larger facility, Pinecrest Health and Fitness, and entered the world of membership-based fitness and Spinning. My gut was telling me that Spinning was going to be big, and we were able to ride that wave starting in 1996. It was Spinning that taught me the power of group fitness. I already had experience with high-end, personal-touch fitness where people paid a lot of money but got a lot for what they paid.

We were profitable and making a comfortable living, but I wanted more. In 2002, I opened Pinecrest Pilates, a small group Pilates studio using reformers. Again I was able to recognize another fitness trend and stay ahead of the curve. Again our Pilates studio was successful and profitable but not at the level that I had always dreamed of.

Two decades of analyzing the fitness industry had sharpened my skill of recognizing big fitness trends, but something was still missing. I had not mastered the business side of things. I was hands-on and personal touch. I was the name and face of each business. I spent so much time teaching, personal training, and working the front desk that I lacked a marketing plan, branding, proper staff training, and recruiting. We were using the wrong software, lacked a sales process, and were just inefficient! Building a reputation and building personal relationships with our members did better than my bottom line.

In 2007, I sold Pinecrest Health and Fitness, continued training my clients, and let my wife run the Pilates studio. I had reached a crossroads. I did not want to give up. I wanted to stay the course. But I still felt like I was playing in the little leagues! I wanted to move up to the big leagues, but I still had not figured out how I would get there.

In 2011, almost 20 years after I started my journey in the fitness profession, I found Orangetheory Fitness. An employee from our equipment maintenance company was working in our Pilates studio when he suddenly had to leave because there was an emergency at Orangetheory Fitness.

Just hearing that name really intrigued me. I went home and Googled it and was blown away by what I learned. As I continued to research the company, I learned that Ellen Latham was its creator. I had been aware of Ellen for years since we both worked in fitness in the South Florida region. I had numerous friends doing Ellen's Ultimate Workout at her studio, and they always raved about how much they loved it.

This all started making sense to me. Twenty years in fitness had earned me one thing for sure—the ability to recognize the next big thing in fitness. I was sure this was it!

The next six months were a struggle, though. Having been my own boss my whole life, I was reluctant to join a franchise whose rules I would have to follow (and that I would pay royalties to). I thought I knew the small group fitness business model and was having trouble justifying the sharing of my gross income with an organization that I thought knew more than it did.

In January 2012, I broke down and signed my first franchise agreement, and the race was on to find a location and build out the studio. We opened our first location, a 2,500-square-foot facility, on October 19, 2012. In our first 11 days of business, our gross income was $20,000 more than my best month at any of my businesses that I had owned in the past 20 years.

I was speechless. I did not think this was real. I figured this was a fluke. The next month we grossed more. Again I was speechless and had trouble believing this was sustainable. Well, after 31 months in operation and increased monthly sales for 31 consecutive months,

I am a huge believer! It still blows my mind, but I am comfortable with it now.

In January 2014 I was fortunate enough to open my second location, a 3,000-square-foot space. We've been in operation for 16 months and this location is even more successful than my first. Now I'm an even bigger believer! We're opening a third location on South Beach in January 2015, with plans to open two more locations in Miami.

This is my twenty-third year in the fitness industry. My dream has come true, and I feel like I am now in the big leagues. Orangetheory Fitness is sweeping across the nation, and I am fortunate enough to have five locations in one of the hottest markets in the country. I have found financial freedom for the first time in my life, and I see a light at the end of the tunnel that I'll one day be able to retire comfortably. And we're taking many more family vacations!

—Mike Singer, Orangetheory franchisee with studios in Florida

I remember meeting Wendy and Erik Skaaleruud—they were positive, upbeat people who couldn't stop smiling! I knew within five minutes that they would hit it out of the park, and they have:

My Orangetheory: I'm Changing People's Lives

There are few moments in your life that you can define as life changing. Marrying my husband, Erik, of 11 years; giving birth to my two boys, Grason and Celyn; and taking my first class at Orangetheory Fitness! Sounds crazy, right?

I have always been a bit of serial entrepreneur, starting my first restaurant business at the age of 22. From there, more restaurants, a landscape business, and a business consulting firm. With each opportunity came a great deal of growth and development; however, I could never prepare myself for what was about to come.

Always on the lookout to diversify my résumé and anxious to find something that spoke to my heart, I was thrilled when Orangetheory Fitness came across my radar four years ago. Erik and I had been working with a few of the founders in multiple capacities over the prior 10 years. Our first business transaction many years back was executed on a handshake. Needless to say, we believed in the integrity behind the team at Orangetheory. Integrity intact, we chose to hop on a plane to get the rest of the story.

We were not disappointed. We spent three days with a total of five people (which I believe was the entire corporate office at the time), worked out with Ellen (and were immediately humbled), and fell in love. On the flight home, I knew not only that I was sold on owning a studio but also that I wanted the entire state of Colorado.

What could have happened in three short days for Erik and I to invest the entire amount of our very tiny life savings, to believe we could rock out a concept that no one in Colorado had heard of, and to be fortunate enough to build a region full of people who fill our hearts every day? It's because I learned years ago to use three levels of measurement when making decisions:

- First, trust my instinct. Instinct is your heart and your gut sending crazy energy through your body. It may scream for you to follow a direction that you may not understand at the time but is absolutely the path to take.
- Second, always do my due diligence. I learned from the Lincoln letter to make sure you have all the facts, write everything down, and give it time to simmer before you act. (President Lincoln wrote a letter to Mrs. Bixby, the mother of five sons serving in the Union army, expressing his condolences for the loss of her five sons—when only one had been killed in battle.)
- Third, and most critical, am I aligning myself with the right people?

Gut? Check. Due diligence? Done. People? No question. We trusted the corporate team and our two partners, Trent and Paig Peaker, who made this possible for us. So we were in.

As with any new venture, we had plenty of growing pains. However, it was so exciting to be part of the growth of a concept we truly believed in. Ironically, the language of Orangetheory seemed to parallel our life—a little Base pace, implementing those things we were comfortable with. Push, getting quite a bit uncomfortable building a business along with a marriage. And All Out, learning to work harder than ever imagined, forcing ourselves out of our box, trusting the greater good, and being challenged to find balance.

To think that I almost passed up this opportunity because I was scared of being involved in a franchise! Orangetheory handed me an incredible business model on a silver platter, and for that I will gladly pay the company's royalty fee! We have a huge support system with franchisees in every market across the United States who experience similar issues and share their problem-solving solutions. The corporate office at Orangetheory has supplied me with templates for employee training and sales processes. The corporate marketing team has allowed me to brand and market in ways I never dreamed possible. We use amazing software and have technologies that we would have never been able to access on our own.

The success we have achieved in just 2.5 years is still hard for me to comprehend, but not a day goes by that I am not grateful for having been afforded this opportunity. And if there was ever to be icing on the cake, I was featured on the cover of a nationally distributed magazine this past month for my success with Orangetheory Fitness. The dream that I had always had of reaching the big leagues had finally happened. I had worked hard, never gave up, and kept that strong work ethic. We stayed the course, and I plan on staying here for the foreseeable future!

What have Erik and I learned the most from the past few years? Each of us has the ability to positively impact the life of someone every day if we so choose. When you give your authentic heart and truly listen to the needs of others, you build an amazing community that thrives on results, companionship, and rewards beyond imagination.

I have learned that I have a power and responsibility as a female owner to nurture, empower, and develop my team every day, which in turn rolls over to our members. The gift of knowing that Erik and I took a risk on a business that ultimately rewards us daily with life-changing stories from every level of our community is the most reward I could ever ask for from living a life of getting comfortable getting uncomfortable.

—Wendy Skaaleruud, Orangetheory franchisee
with studios in Colorado

The last franchisee featured in this chapter, Terry Blachek, was already a seasoned fitness professional when he first got involved with Orangetheory in 2010. He's been with us since Orangetheory's first year and was instrumental in developing our Splat logo, developing our presale programs, and helping our franchisees strive for excellence. I still remember him telling me early on, "Ellen, we have something *big* here."

My Orangetheory:
It's Your Team That Makes the Difference

In February 2010, I heard about Ellen's and the Ultimate Workout. I invited my friend Dave Hardy to check out the studio and learn more about it. At the time, I had 25+ years of health club experience and had been consulting with health clubs around the world. After meeting Ellen and watching a class or two, I talked to my wife about it, and we decided to try the workout ourselves. I learned from Ellen that she was talking to Dave Long and Jerome Kern about franchising the concept. I'd worked with Dave before and wound up consulting for them to help build the company's sales systems and sales manuals.

Several months later, I invested in the company to become an initial partner. I also purchased the west coast of Florida and opened my first Orangetheory studio in St. Petersburg in February 2011. It was the fifth Orangetheory studio to open and the first to do a presale, where we sold memberships before the studio was up and running. I opened studios in St. Petersburg and Tampa and started a concept called the 500 Club, where a new studio strives to attain 500 members within 30 days of opening. Since then I've opened studios in Texas and now own 16 studios.

People have asked me what my secret sauce is, and it's the people you hire. It's finding, recruiting, training, mentoring, coaching, and believing in them. In turn, they believe in me and our young, emerging brand. I've found a new family, and they have found me. Orangetheory is someone and something to believe in; something to get excited about and believe in; and something that provides purpose in their life and has created a career for them. The greatest gift we receive is the ability to change people's lives—we are truly making a difference in the lives of people in the community we serve.

The boutique concept has become a trend in the health club industry. So many people in the past seven years have been focused on budget clubs and low-price models of $10 per month. OTF is the opposite and filled a void—the void was a sense of belonging, a sense of community, a culture, a family, versus going into a big box, saying "Hi" and "Good-bye," and using the equipment. Orangetheory takes a personal interest in members and guests, uses their names, provides personal service, and is an affordable way to get a trainer. Orangetheory provides a coach, music, and friends at an affordable rate of $10–$16 per workout. Pretty cool, right?

Over the past five and a half years, I've learned that:

- Sometimes you just have to go with what you got and what you believe in and trust that others will believe in it also.
- The relationships outweigh the money.

- I didn't know everything about the fitness business, and despite how long I had been in it, this was a little different.
- After I liquidated my entire 401(K) and bought in, there was no turning back, and I needed to find a way to win and a way to make it work. And we did.
- The people you surround yourself with are the key to your success. You cannot do it alone, and I am truly indebted to Troy Taylor, Josh Whisman, and Abdul Fox for their belief in me and for allowing me to lead.
- You cannot always do it on your own. I would not be in the position I am today if Edgar Corona had not believed in me and became my partner to open studios in the Tampa market.
- I need to believe in myself but believe in my team more than me. They took me further than I ever could have taken myself.
- The collective wisdom of the group and idea sharing and coming up with a plan together—going through adversity or the crucible of presales—are what bring teams together. And that sometimes you need a guy like Paul Reuter at Orangetheory corporate who is around to vent and tell your frustrations to.

Finally, I am grateful for Dave Hardy for professional guidance, for Dave Long and Jerome Kern for seeing further than any of us did in the beginning, and for Ellen. The passion that woman has is second to none. You can see it in her eyes when she talks about her dad and the picture she had of him in her studio. I am grateful for her in the concept and her dedication to sharing it with the world.

—Terry Blachek, franchisee with studios in Florida and Texas

Aren't these stories inspiring? I am personally inspired by the Orangetheory franchisees I've met and have found that like me, they are committed to excellence and to continual improvement. They Push themselves just like we Push ourselves at Orangetheory. My ideal franchisee is someone who's willing to come out of Base and Push to create All Out results in their business. And if that sounds like you, consider whether franchising might be a good fit for you!

9

What's Next? Using Your Extra Oxygen

From reading this book, you now know that I've been in the fitness industry for nearly four decades. Yet I haven't worked a day in my life!

I was reminded of this when I spoke with my 27-year-old son, Evan, yesterday. He's now co-owner of two Orangetheory Fitness studios in Florida and Tennessee. He's in the presales stage at his second studio and was thrilled to report his presales numbers to me. I could hear the excitement and energy coming through the phone! Evan told me he'd worked four weeks straight, averaging 12 hours a day, without a day off! Then he added, "You know, Ma, it doesn't feel like you're working when you love what you do!"

Well, yeah! I know just how he feels. I've been saying the same thing since I started in this business. I have dedicated my life to be a leader in fitness and help others change their I Can't channels to I Can by **focusing on what they have instead of what they don't have**. I love making the impossible possible for people! While doing so, I've helped others and helped myself become the best version of myself. I use that phrase a lot because I really try to live by that—I'm always striving to be the best version of me I can be.

That means I'm not just the creator of Orangetheory—I'm a member, too! This morning, I completed a great Orangetheory endurance workout. I was feeling strong and rested, so I took my Base, Push, and All Out up by 0.5 mph. I left feeling energized and accomplished. I definitely consumed more oxygen today, both during my workout and afterward!

I plan to do the same in my life. I will pay attention to days that I feel stronger and more rested and Push a little harder. I will also give myself active recovery time after those Pushes so I can refuel to successfully pursue another Push. As you've seen in this book, the lessons of Base/Push/All Out apply both inside the Orangetheory studio and outside of it! The ability to consume more oxygen also gives me the ability to be the best version of me.

How do you use your extra oxygen? That will depend on where you're at in your life and what your priorities are. In my 20s, I used to my oxygen to look, feel, and move at the highest level I could. I did 10K races, triathlons, and aerobic challenges. In my 30s, most of my oxygen was used to raise my son, Evan. He was my biggest priority. In my 40s, I was increasing my number of breathless moments by putting bigger expectations on myself. I started challenging myself in new ways—like opening Ellen's and creating the Ultimate Workout.

Now, I'm in my 50s (I turn 59 next month), and I will continue to Push and go All Out, blowing up those mitochondria, the power plants in my cells. That means continuing to be active and disciplined and continuing to get my Orange on, which will ensure a sufficient oxygen supply to keep me moving forward. I know there is room for more growth—for new Pushes and All Outs. I will continue to see possibilities and new meaning in my life and profession.

I will also continue to learn because that's my personal fuel that feeds my spirit. Learning keeps me energized and oxygenated. I believe complacency happens when you run low on oxygen, and I will not let that happen. I don't want to be complacent! People have said to me, "So, Ellen, are you going to take it easy now?"

In a word, no! I intend to continue to challenge myself, to learn, and to grow. I'm going to capitalize on this large volume of oxygen to pursue motivational public speaking, nationally and internationally. I want to make a difference with people I may never be able to meet personally but can have a positive impact on in other ways. I want to help other women, single parents, and business entrepreneurs to understand how and when to Push and reach for some All Outs!

Yes, oxygen is essential for this. But I've also given myself permission to dream big and take calculated risks. That kind of challenge continues to build my success muscle. And I hope this book will help you do the same, no matter what obstacles may seem to stand in your way.

My dad was my first, and most important, role model in my life. While still athletic and strong in his 60s, he was eventually diagnosed with Parkinson's disease. Yet that didn't change his outlook. He still focused on what he had, not what was being taken away from him. He was always upbeat and positive and loved to spend time with his family, especially his four grandsons, right up until his last years when he was crippled and confined to a wheelchair, unable to move. He died at 78 years of age.

I always thought it was so strange that such an active, vital man would get a disease that takes away your physical body and the ability to move. (Parkinson's stops the secretion of dopamine in the brain, which is needed to maintain movement.) But even after he passed, my father left behind an abundance of oxygen in the air. How? Because he changed the lives of his family and literally thousands of the students he taught and coached.

My dad made it possible for me to live a legacy. Every day, I try to use his internal strength and share it with Orangetheory members and employees. When negative thoughts creep up, I think of my father and his focus on gratitude for what he had—and how he made the most of his own oxygen. I have always believed that some of my own oxygen came from my dad. I hope that I'll be able to leave oxygen for those I care about one day as well.

But for now, I'm going to use that oxygen to embrace the gratitude I feel. I cannot put into words the feeling I have when I reflect on the positive effects my workouts have had on many people worldwide who have done them. I am humbled and grateful for all the people who have trusted me to help them change that I Can't channel to I Can and to become the best physical versions of themselves. So I would like to say thank you!

Finally, I leave you with a challenge. This book is called *Push: The Keys to Living an All Out Life*. If you're dissatisfied with something in your life, I challenge you to look at your fitness program—and your life—and *choose* to live beyond Base. Choose to Push. Push yourself at Orangetheory and in your life. I guarantee you will end up with more oxygen—and more All Out moments.

Get in Touch

Are you an Orangetheory member? A franchisee? An employee? I would love to hear *your* story and how Orangetheory has affected you. Please e-mail me at the address below.

And if you haven't yet experienced the Orangetheory Fitness workout, I encourage you to use the two complimentary passes included with this book! Grab a friend, and try the class to find your Base, Push, and physical and personal All Out.

Here's to becoming the best physical version of *you*.

Ellen Latham
elatham@orangetheoryfitness.com

Appendix: Selected Research

Akca, F. "Prediction of rowing ergometer performance from functional anaerobic power, strength and anthropometric components." *Journal of Human Kinetics* 41 (July 8, 2014): 133–142.

Bahr, R. "Excess post-exercise oxygen consumption—magnitude, mechanisms and practical implications." *Acta Physiologica Scandinavica Supplementum* 605 (1993): 1–70.

Bahr, R., A. T. Høstmark, E. A. Newsholme, O. Grønnerød, and O. M. Sejersted. "Effect of exercise on recovery changes in plasma levels of FFA, glycerol, glucose and catecholamines." *Acta Physiologica Scandinavica* 143, no. 1 (September 1991): 105–115.

Bielinski, R., Y. Schutz, and E. Jäquier. "Energy metabolism during the postexercise recovery in man." *American Journal of Clinical Nutrition* 42, no. 1 (July 1985): 69–82.

Børsheim, E., and R. Bahr. "Effect of exercise intensity, duration and mode on post-exercise oxygen consumption." *Sports Medicine* 33, no. 14 (2005): 1037–1060.

Boutcher, S. H. "High-intensity intermittent exercise and fat loss." *Journal of Obesity* 2011 (2011): 868305.

Buchheit, M., P. B. Laursen, and S. Ahmaidi. "Parasympathetic reactivation after repeated sprint exercise." *American Journal of Physiology* 293, no. 1 (2007): H133–H141.

Burgomaster, K. A., K. R. Howarth, S. M. Phillips, et al. "Similar metabolic adaptations during exercise after low volume sprint interval and traditional endurance training in humans." *Journal of Physiology* 84, no. 1 (2008): 151–160.

Christmass, M. A., B. Dawson, and P. G. Arthur. "Effect of work and recovery duration on skeletal muscle oxygenation and fuel use during sustained intermittent exercise." *European Journal of Applied Physiology and Occupational Physiology* 80, no. 5 (1999): 436–447.

Dudley, G. A., W. M. Abraham, and R. L. Terjung. "Influence of exercise intensity and duration on biochemical adaptations in skeletal muscle." *Journal of Applied Physiology: Respiratory, Environmental, and Exercise Physiology* 53, no. 4 (October 1982): 844–850.

Gibala, M. "Molecular responses to high-intensity interval exercise." *Applied Physiology, Nutrition, and Metabolism* 34, no. 3 (2009): 428–432.

Gibala, M. J., and S. L. McGee. "Metabolic adaptations to short-term high-intensity interval training: a little pain for a lot of gain?" *Exercise and Sport Sciences Reviews* 36, no. 20 (2008): 58–63.

Gibala, M. J., S. L. McGee, A. P. Garnham, K. F. Howlett, R. J. Snow, and M. Hargreaves. "Brief intense interval exercise activates AMPK and p38 MAPK signaling and increases the expression of PGC-1 in human skeletal muscle." *Journal of Applied Physiology* 106, no. 3 (2009): 929–934.

Godfrey, R. J., Z. Madgwick, and G. P. Whyte. "The exercise-induced growth hormone response in athletes." *Sports Medicine* 33, no. 8 (2003): 599–613.

Helgerud, J., K. Høydal, E. Wang, et al. "Aerobic high-intensity intervals improve VO_2 max more than moderate training." *Medicine and Science in Sports and Exercise* 39, no. 4 (2007): 665–671.

Hickson, R. C., and M. A. Rosenkotter. "Separate turnover of cytochrome c and myoglobin in the red types of skeletal muscle." *American Journal of Physiology* 241, no. 3 (September 1981): C140–C144.

Horn, P., P. Ostadal, and B. Ostadal. "Rowing increases stroke volume and cardiac output to a greater extent than cycling." *Physiological Research* 64, no. 2 (May 20, 2015): 203–207.

Laforgia, J., R. T. Withers, and C. J. Gore. "Effects of exercise intensity and duration on the excess post-exercise oxygen consumption." *Journal of Sports Sciences* 24, no. 12 (2006): 1247–1264.

LaRocca, T. J., D. R. Seals, and G. L. Pierce. "Leukocyte telomere length is preserved with aging in endurance exercise-trained adults and related to maximal capacity." *Mechanics of Ageing and Development* 131, no. 2 (February 2010): 165–167.

Little, J. P., A. Safdar, N. Cermak, M. A. Tarnopolsky, and M. J. Gibala. "Acute endurance exercise increases the nuclear abundance of PGC-1 alpha in trained human skeletal muscle." *American Journal of Physiology* 298, no. 4 (2010): R912–R917.

Macdougall, J. D., A. L. Hicks, J. R. Macdonald, R. S. Mckelvie, H. J. Green, and K. M. Smith. "Muscle performance and enzymatic adaptations to sprint interval training." *Journal of Applied Physiology* 84, no. 6 (1998): 2138–2142.

Nevill, M. E., D. J. Holmyard, G. M. Hall, et al. "Growth hormone responses to treadmill sprinting in spring- and endurance-trained athletes." *European Journal of Applied Physiology and Occupational Physiology* 72, no. 5–6 (1996): 460–467.

Perry, C. G. R., G. J. F. Heigenhauser, A. Bonen, and L. L. Spriet. "High-intensity aerobic interval training increases fat and carbohydrate metabolic capacities in human skeletal muscle." *Applied Physiology, Nutrition, and Metabolism* 33, no. 6 (2008): 1112–1123.

Rebuffe-Scrive, M., B. Anderson, L. Olbe, and P. Pjorntorp. "Metabolism of adipose tissue in intra-abdominal deposits of nonobese men and women." *Metabolism* 38, no. 5 (1989): 453–458.

Riviere, D., F. Crampes, M. Beauville, and M. Garrigues. "Lipolytic response of fat cells to catecholamines in sedentary and exercise-trained women." *Journal of Applied Psychology* 66, no. 1 (1989): 330–335.

Schuenke, M. D., R. P. Mikat, and J. M. McBride. "Effect of an acute period of resistance exercise on excess post-exercise oxygen consumption: implications for body mass management." *European Journal of Applied Physiology* 86, no. 5 (March 2002): 411–417.

Scott, C. B., A. Croteau, and T. Ravlo. "Energy expenditure before, during, and after the bench press." *Journal of Strength and Conditioning Research* 23, no. 2 (March 2009): 611–618.

Scott, C. B., and R. B. Kemp. "Direct and indirect calorimetry of lactate oxidation: implications for whole-body energy expenditure." *Journal of Sports Sciences* 23, no. 1 (January 2005): 15–19.

Tabata, I., K. Nishimura, and M. Kouzaki, et al. "Effects of moderate-intensity endurance and high-intensity intermittent training on anaerobic capacity and VO$_2$ max." *Medicine and Science in Sports and Exercise* 28, no. 10 (1996): 1327–1330.

Talanian, J. L., S. D. R. Galloway, J. G. F. Heigenhauser, A. Bonen, and L. L. Spriet. "Two weeks of high-intensity aerobic interval training increases the capacity for fat oxidation during exercise in women." *Journal of Applied Physiology* 102, no. 4 (2007): 1439–1447.

Teixeira, P. J., S. B. Going, L. B. Houtkooper, et al. "Pretreatment predictors of attrition and successful weight management in women." *International Journal of Obesity* 28, no. 9 (2004): 1124–1133.

Tonoli, C., E. Heyman, L. Buyse, B. Roelands, M. F. Piacentini, S. Bailey, N. Pattyn, S. Berthoin, and R. Meeusen. "Neurotrophins and cognitive functions in T1D compared with healthy controls: effects of a high-intensity exercise." *Applied Physiology and Nutritional Metabolism* 40, no. 1 (January 2015): 20–27.

Trapp, E. G., D. J. Chisholm, and S. H. Boutcher. "Metabolic response of trained and untrained women during high-intensity intermittent cycle exercise." *American Journal of Physiology* 293, no. 6 (2007): R2370–R2375.

Trapp, E. G., D. J. Chisholm, J. Freund, and S. H. Boutcher. "The effects of high-intensity intermittent exercise training on fat loss and fasting insulin levels of young women." *International Journal of Obesity* 32, no. 40 (2008): 684–691.

Tremblay, A., J.-A. Simoneau, and C. Bouchard. "Impact of exercise intensity on body fatness and skeletal muscle metabolism." *Metabolism* 43, no. 7 (1994): 814–818.

Vuorimaa, T., M. Ahotupa, K. Häkkinen, and T. Vasankari. "Different hormonal response to continuous and intermittent exercise in middle-distance and marathon runners." *Scandinavian Journal of Medicine and Science in Sports* 18, no. 5 (2008): 565–572.

Whyte, L. J., M. R. Gill, and A. J. Cathcart. "Effect of 2 weeks of sprint interval training on health-related outcomes in sedentary overweight/obese men." *Metabolism Clinical and Experimental* 59, no. 10 (2010): 1421–1428.

Zouhal, H., C. Jacob, P. Delamarche, and A. Gratas-Delamarche. "Catecholamines and the effects of exercise, training and gender." *Sports Medicine* 38, no. 5 (2008): 401–423.

About the Author

Author Ellen Latham, MS, is a highly trained physiologist with a life-long passion for health and fitness and four decades of experience in the

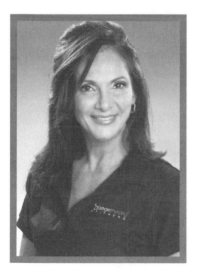

fitness industry. She grew up in Niagara Falls, New York, and was inspired by her father, Arthur Calandrelli, a popular physical education teacher and high school football coach, to choose a career in fitness. She holds a bachelor's degree in physical education and a master's degree in exercise physiology from the State University of New York at Buffalo.

Using her education, training, experience, and knowledge, she created and launched the cutting-edge Ultimate Workout in 2009. The Ultimate Workout became the foundation for Orangetheory Fitness, one of the fastest-growing fitness franchises in the world.

Before perfecting her signature workout, Ellen was an exercise physiologist and manager at well-known spas in the Miami/Fort Lauderdale area. She opened the first group equipment-based Pilates studio in Florida in 2000 in Fort Lauderdale. Ellen has worked as a personal trainer to celebrities, appeared as a fitness expert on national television networks, and written for a number of print publications.

Ellen is a partner and founder of Orangetheory Fitness and owner of Ellen's Ultimate Workout studio in Fort Lauderdale. She is also a motivational speaker who strives to help people learn how to Push in their lives to become the best versions of themselves.

Ellen lives with her partner, Nick Granteed, in Fort Lauderdale. Her adult son, Evan Latham, co-owns two Orangetheory Fitness studios in Florida and Tennessee.